THE
THAI MASSAGE
MANUAL

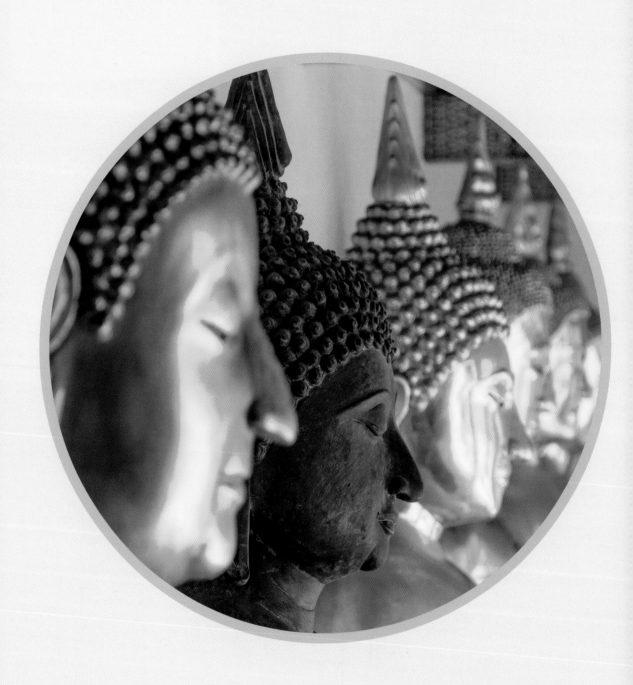

MARIA MERCATI

PHOTOGRAPHY BY SUE ATKINSON

THE THAI MASSAGE MANUAL

NATURAL THERAPY FOR FLEXIBILITY, RELAXATION AND ENERGY BALANCE

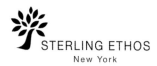

STERLING ETHOS
New York

To my loving family:
Trevor, Gisela, Gina, Graham and Danella.

PLEASE NOTE
This book is not intended as guidance for the diagnosis or treatment of serious health problems; please refer to a medical professional if you are in any doubt about any aspect of a person's condition. Please note pregnant women should not be treated with Thai massage. The author and publisher cannot be held responsible for any injuries that may result from the use of information in this book.

STERLING ETHOS and the distinctive Sterling Ethos logo are registered trademarks of Sterling Publishing Co., Inc.

Text copyright © 1998, 2017 by Maria Mercati
Photographs copyright © 1998, 2017 by Sue Atkinson
Illustrations copyright © 1998, 2017 by Joanna Cameron
This edition copyright © 2017 by Eddison Books Limited
www.eddisonbooks.com

ISBN 978-1-4549-2856-0

Distributed in Canada by Sterling Publishing
c/o Canadian Manda Group, 664 Annette Street
Toronto, Ontario, Canada M6S 2C8

For information about custom editions, special sales, premium and corporate purchases, please contact Sterling Special Sales at 800-805-5489 or specialsales@sterlingpublishing.com.

Manufactured in China

10 9 8 7 6 5 4 3 2 1

www.sterlingpublishing.com

CONTENTS

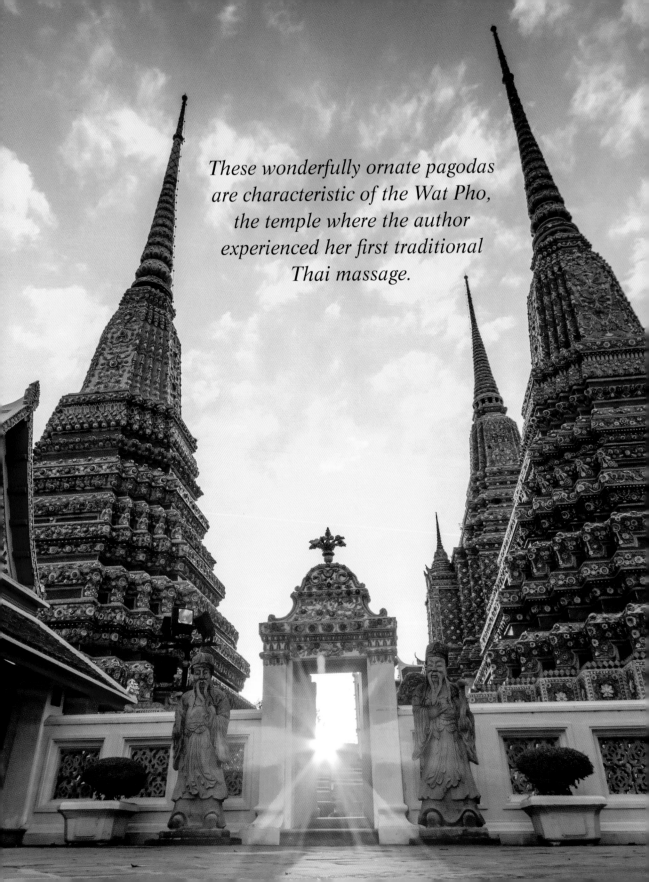

*These wonderfully ornate pagodas
are characteristic of the Wat Pho,
the temple where the author
experienced her first traditional
Thai massage.*

A NOTE FROM THE AUTHOR

M. B. Mercati.

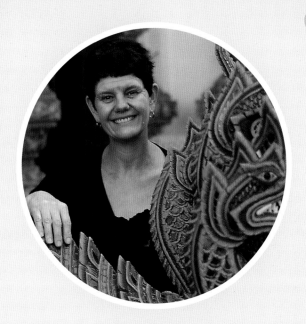

During the early 1980s I lived with my family in Indonesia for four years. It was here that I first discovered the healing massage. Extensive travels in Southeast Asia eventually brought me to Thailand, where I began treatment and training in traditional Thai massage. Since childhood I had suffered from Perthes disease – a chronic degenerative condition of the hip joint – and the wonderful stretching effects of Thai massage seemed like a miracle cure. Flexibility in my legs, including the affected joint, improved enormously, and Thai massage has continued to enhance the flexibility and mobility of my body to the present day. However, Thai massage not only balances the body's need for movement and stretching, it also produces powerful feelings of well-being and happiness.

My interest in oriental medicine was so aroused that I also undertook to study Tui Na Chinese massage and acupuncture in China. After several visits to China, I subsequently returned to Thailand to study Thai massage at the sacred Wat Pho temple in Bangkok and the Old Medicine Hospital in Chiang Mai. I also received private tuition from Chaiyuth Priyasith, one of Thailand's most respected masters.

SPREADING THE WORD

To give others the opportunity to experience these ancient, yet thriving oriental therapies, I established the Bodyharmonics® Centre in Cheltenham, England, in 1993. Training and treatment in Thai bodywork and Indonesian traditional massage, Tui Na Chinese massage and acupuncture are provided there. Today, all the members of my family share my passion for traditional oriental bodywork. I believe that Thai traditional massage reaches those parts of the body and mind that other forms of massage fail to reach, and I hope that by reading this book you too will be motivated to try it and experience its unique benefits yourself.

This manual will help you to discover healing benefits of Thai massage for yourself, your friends and family.

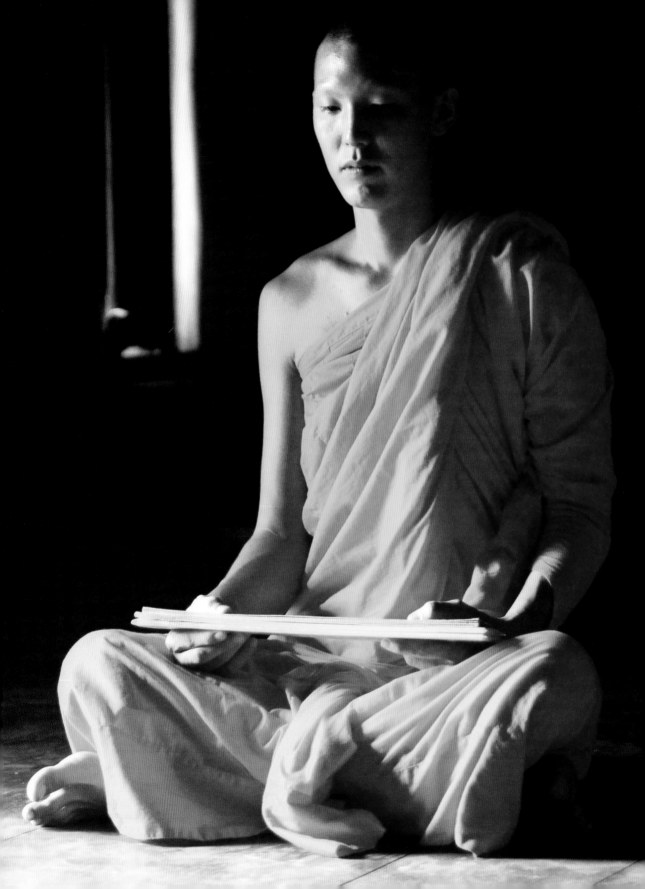

INTRODUCTION

นวดไทยโบราณ

Nuad Boran means 'Traditional Thai Massage'

Thai massage is one of the ancient healing arts of traditional Thai medicine – the others are herbal medicine and spiritual meditation. The term 'massage' conjures up images of something quite different from Thai massage, which, even at its most basic, is a complex sequence of soft tissue pressing, stretching, twisting and joint manipulations. For this reason, rather than 'massage', we prefer to use the term 'Thai bodywork', which is used frequently throughout the book.

Thai bodywork has been in a process of constant evolution for over 1,000 years. It's not surprising, therefore, to find many subtle variations in the techniques used by different practitioners, and even greater differences are apparent between the styles of bodywork characteristic of the north and south of Thailand. The techniques presented by Maria Mercati in this book are essentially a potpourri of those taken from various regions of the country. Beginners will find them flowing and harmonious and very similar to what you could expect to receive at the hands of a Thai master.

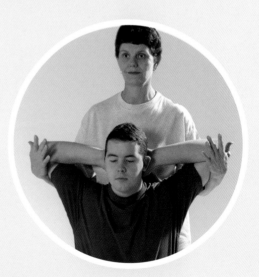

Maria Mercati performs a butterfly shoulder stretch on her son, Graham (see page 143).

TRADITIONAL THAI MASSAGE

Traditional Thai massage has been practised in more or less its present form for at least 1,000 years. It's a member of the whole family of oriental bodywork, based on the intrinsic energy flow and energy balance theory of health and healing. Other family members include Tui Na Chinese, Ayurvedic Indian and Shiatsu Japanese massage. Thai massage is rooted in Ayurvedic medicine, which arrived in Thailand over 2,000 years ago. Thai stretching techniques make the Indian yogic influence obvious.

Ayurvedic and Chinese Medicine have mapped the energy networks of the body. Ayurvedic and Thai massage historically refer to 72,000 theoretical lines, called Sen. As a guide to the therapist, Thai massage uses ten Sen lines, which are based on drawings from the Wat Pho tablets. Chinese Medicine has fourteen lines, or meridians, that were already documented 2,300 years ago.

The first recorded Western commentary on Thai medicine was made in 1690 by Simon de la Loubère, a French diplomat, who observed: 'When any person is sick at Siam he begins with causing his whole body to be moulded by one who is skilful herein, who gets upon the body of the sick person and tramples him under his feet.'

THE ROLE OF THAI MASSAGE

Who needs traditional Thai massage and manipulation? You do, if your body is crying out: 'Touch me', 'Stretch me', 'Squeeze me', 'Hold me', 'Listen to me', 'Comfort me' or 'Heal me'. Such body cries often go unheard. This book will help you to discover how Thai bodywork can answer your body's pleas, and it could be the first important step that leads you to seek its unique benefits.

Modern lifestyles are often dominated by the desire to achieve independence and fulfilment through the use of machinery and new technology. We aim to make our lives easy and convenient and, with ever more leisure time, hope that we will be healthy, youthful and pain-free enough to enjoy life. There's a distinct trend towards overindulgence, and this, unfortunately, goes hand in hand with increasing deprivation in areas such as regular exercise and interaction with others on a caring and compassionate level. This book is written in the firm belief that Thai bodywork involves just such an interaction, enabling you to share with another person in a mutual 'un-Thai-ing' of physical and emotional knots. Interaction through physical contact has been fundamental to most Eastern cultures for thousands of years, yet the practice still remains quite foreign to most Westerners.

It should be emphasized that traditional Thai massage is not the same thing as the media-sensationalized activities that take place in massage parlours throughout the tourist centres of Thailand. It's not about sexual gratification but about wholeness, balance, health and happiness. Thai massage means togetherness at a physical level, quite outside the sexual, and is, for all of us, one of the vital components of a happy, balanced life.

TRADITIONAL THAI ORIGINS

Like the origin of the Thai people, the history of traditional Thai massage is obscure. Thailand was at the crossroads of the ancient migration routes that saw waves of civilizations and cultures passing through. The combination of Thailand's closeness to China and its position on one of the main trade routes from India has resulted in many cultural and religious influences, particularly Buddhism, being brought to bear on its early inhabitants.

Folk tradition credits Jivaka Kumar Bhaccha, also known as Shivago Komparaj, as the founder

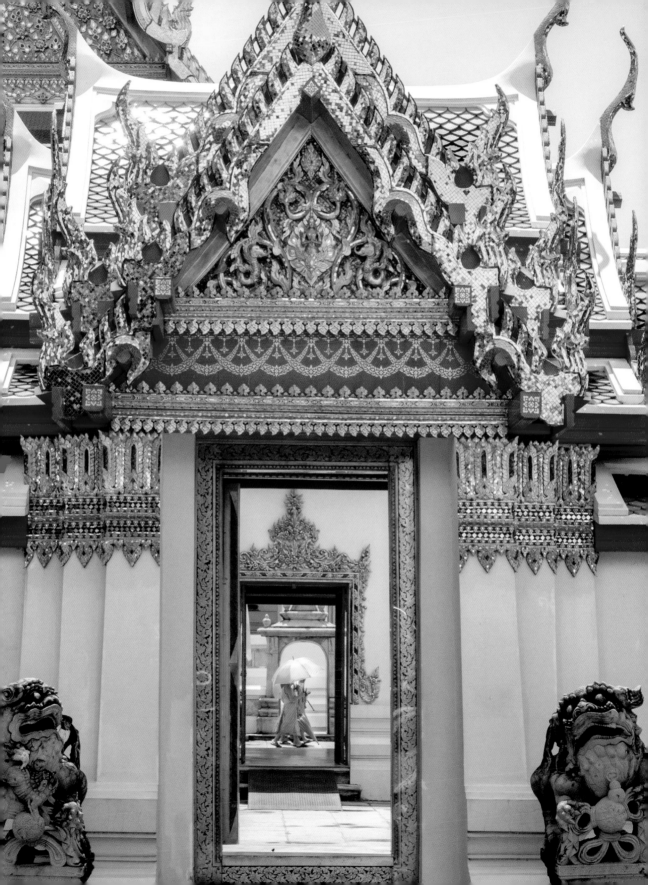

of Thai massage. A friend and physician to the Buddha some 2,500 years ago, he is still revered as the 'father of Thai medicine'. None of the information regarding massage procedures was written down and it was passed by word of mouth from generation to generation. Medical texts that included detailed descriptions of Thai massage, as it was then practised, were eventually recorded in the Pali language on palm leaves. These were venerated as religious texts and held in safe keeping in the old capital city of Ayutthaya. During the eighteenth century Ayutthaya was overrun by Burmese invaders, and many of the precious texts were destroyed. In 1832, King Rama III had all the surviving texts carved in stone as descriptive epigraphs at Wat Pho, Bangkok's largest temple.

WAT PHO TEMPLE

'Wats' are temples or monasteries. Besides being focal points for the practice of Buddhism, the Wats have always provided for the health needs of the people. The Wat Pho is the most famous of them. It dates back to the sixteenth century and houses the famous reclining Buddha, which is 46 metres (150 feet) long and 15 metres (49 feet) high, together with the largest collection of Buddha images in Thailand. There are sixty carved epigraphs that depict the ten Sen lines and pressure points and embody all the information from the Pali texts that still survived during the reign of Rama III. Outside the temple is a collection of stone statues that shows various classical Thai massage techniques. Wat Pho is the national centre for the teaching and preservation of traditional Thai medicine. Most Thais are Buddhists and even today are devoted to Buddha's teachings of non-violence, loving kindness and compassion. Monks are still supported by gifts of food, and making regular offerings at the temples is regarded as virtuous. With origins rooted in Buddhist philosophy, it's no surprise that traditional Thai

massage, for much of its history, has been seen as a religious rite. Until quite recently, Thai massage was only officially practised by monks, so precluding women as potential recipients. Various forms of folk massage were, and still are, practised within families, with family members massaging one another.

THE SEN LINES

In this book, sections of the Chinese Meridians are used where they correspond to similar positions of the Thai Sen lines. They can be described and located much more accurately than the Sen lines.

The body's vital life energy flows along these Meridians and powers all physical, mental and emotional processes. The Chinese call this energy 'Qi', and the Indians call it 'Prana'. Any imbalance or blockage in the distribution of this energy can cause pain and disease. When the system is working well and energy distribution is balanced, you feel happy, relaxed, energetic and free from stiffness and pain.

The application of pressure along these Sen/Meridians helps to release any energy blockages. Pressing and stretching muscles makes them more receptive to this flow. In chapter 3 of this book each lesson begins with a diagram of the Sen/Meridians to guide your pressing as you massage the relevant section of the body. In addition, dots and arrows are superimposed over the photographs of many of the techniques so that you can see clearly the direction and the full range of movement involved in all the manipulations.

WHAT THAI BODYWORK CAN DO

Yoga is an effective way of remaining healthy and flexible. Receiving Thai bodywork, however, is the ultimate lazy and simple way of obtaining all the benefits of yoga and more – without having to do it yourself.

These are two of the descriptive epigraphs that were etched in stone by order of King Rama III. The complete series can be seen at Wat Pho and represents all the surviving ancient texts on Thai traditional massage.

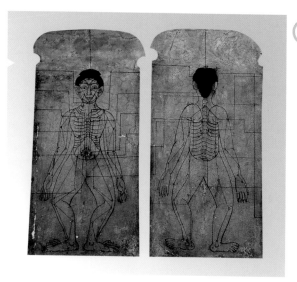

You'll be guided towards mastering a comprehensive range of Thai massage and manipulation techniques, presenting you with a flowing sequence that can help to maintain a youthful body. The techniques can also be used as a healing treatment for chronic pain (see chapter 4).

Stiffness and loss of flexibility are regarded as the inevitable result of the ageing process in the Western world. How you feel – physically, mentally and emotionally – is more important than your mere physical age. Thai bodywork is unique in its ability to preserve youthfulness.

THE SECRET OF THAI BODYWORK

Thai bodywork enables you to press your muscles and thereby balance energy levels. This is what affects flexibility and equalizes the effects of muscles on both sides of the body. The amount of movement a muscle can produce at a joint is determined by the difference between its length when relaxed and when fully contracted. When muscles are tense, they become shorter, even when you aren't consciously contracting them. This can happen through overworking them or by not using them enough, or it could be due to emotional tension. Whatever the cause, the end result is progressively more restricted movement and the onset of stiffness, aches and pains, which are all characteristic of the ageing process.

Muscles that shorten and become tense can create uneven forces on the spine – that all-important container of the spinal cord. This, in turn, creates the back pain, neck pain and headaches

that can so easily become a regular feature of daily life. With their unique ability to stretch all the most important muscles in the body systematically, Thai manipulations enable you to achieve effects that are unlike those of any other bodywork.

You should not see Thai bodywork as a mere physical experience. Indeed, if that is all it turns out to be, then it has largely failed to achieve its real potential. The giving and receiving of Thai bodywork is an ideal way of providing for the subtle yet powerful interchange of intrinsic energy between two individuals. It's always a two-way process, and achievement depends on the caring and compassionate way in which it is given. Even in this day and age, Thai bodywork is a vital necessity for everyday life because it underpins health and well-being. It's the perfect vehicle for two people to come together with a view to attaining this mutual balancing of energy and life force. Thai bodywork embodies all the harmony and rhythm often lacking in our lives.

THAI BODYWORK IN PRACTICE

The many techniques used in Thai bodywork are all designed to facilitate and stimulate the flow of intrinsic energies and to release blockages that would otherwise preclude the attainment of balance that's essential for maintaining a healthy, pain-free body. In this context, 'healthy' and 'pain-free' refer not only to the purely physical but also to the mental, emotional and spiritual aspects of your being.

In this book you'll find more than 150 different techniques that can be used in a massage. Feet, palms, thumbs, elbows and knees are all used to apply deep pressure along the Sen. Other, quite different, techniques are used to apply twists and stretches, and these resemble a kind of applied yoga. At all times the pace is measured and unhurried. When moving from one technique to the next, the movement should be rhythmical, flowing, harmonious and smooth.

Thai bodywork starts in the supine position – lying on the back – and then each side is worked. This is followed by the prone position – lying face downwards – and the sequence finishes in the sitting position. This routine always begins with the feet, which are subjected to a variety of presses, stretches and flexion that would surprise even a reflexologist! The legs are systematically positioned through a range of postures that present the energy channels to their best advantage.

However, it's the manipulations for which Thai bodywork is renowned. These are designed to stretch every accessible muscle just a little more than it would normally be stretched under the action of strongly contracting antagonistic muscles. In the process, all the principal joints are likewise moved just a little more than when they are operating under their own muscle power.

TOUCH ME, STRETCH ME
Touch is one of the greatest medicines. It soothes, releases and comforts us. Our wholeness is nourished by frequent and regular doses of this all-pervading medicine.

Wholeness, in this context, includes spiritual and emotional aspects as well as the more

easily observed physical ones. When looked at with a knowledge of Western medicine, it's easy to see how massage and manipulation can stimulate the flow of blood and lymph (tissue fluid), warm the tissues, improve flexibility and ease pain, all of which are essentially physical.

Such is the power of touch that it also reaches far into the hidden recesses of our being. It has been shown that touch can result in the release of chemical substances within the nervous system called endorphins, which counteract pain and produce a strong feeling of well-being.

Thai bodywork involves different forms of touch – pressing, stretching and twisting – which have been honed to perfection over the ages. Those who receive Thai bodywork regularly will experience feelings of relaxation, peace of mind, happiness, flexibility and youthfulness.

HEAL ME
The word 'heal' suggests ill health or disease, but its meaning in the context of this book requires a much wider definition of health than is commonly recognized. Health is not just physical well-being or general lack of disease; it is a statement regarding the balance that exists between all those factors that contribute to our sense of 'wholeness', both internal and external. Health, though difficult to define in any accurate, all-embracing way, is nevertheless characterized by feelings of vitality, flexibility, freedom from pain, contentment and a sense of wholeness.

The healthy person has, above all else, a balance in their life. One of the adverse spin-offs from life lived in the fast lane is a disturbance of this balance, and when this happens you must have time and space in which to restore that elusive equilibrium. Sharing Thai bodywork with a partner or receiving it from a qualified practitioner are certainly some of the most effective means of doing this.

STAY YOUNG, STAY HEALTHY

Pain is the biggest single obstacle to happiness, and pain of any kind, at any level, is a reflection of imbalance. This results from too much of some things and not enough of others. The body will experience pain if, for example, it has too much rich food or too much violent exercise. But pains of no less a magnitude will be experienced if insufficient food is eaten and no exercise is taken. Pain will also be experienced when the desires of the mind remain unfulfilled, but equally intense pain will be felt when desire is so restricted that there is no driving force for any progress.

The quest for health should be regarded as the search for balance in every facet of our lives. Rest and relaxation are wonderful ways of calming the mind and body to help the balancing process that we commonly call 'healing'; and there are many things we can do in our daily lives to help to make it happen. Receiving Thai bodywork is one of them. Simultaneously, Thai bodywork can give a sublimely rhythmical workout that perfectly balances the body's need for movement and stretching, while also providing a relaxed state in which excessive worry and desire simply seem to evaporate.

'THE FOUR DIVINE STATES OF CONSCIOUSNESS'

As mentioned earlier, traditional Thai massage was originally practised in Buddhist temples because of its religious significance. It was regarded as one of the many ways of working towards the 'Four Divine States of Consciousness', which for Buddhists are a necessary prerequisite for complete happiness. The qualities embodied in these states are:

- Metta: *the desire to make others happy and the ability to show loving kindness.*
- Karuna: *compassion for all who suffer and a desire to ease their sufferings.*
- Mudita: *rejoicing with those who have good fortune and never feeling envy.*
- Upekkha: *regarding your fellows without prejudice or preference.*

From the Buddhist viewpoint, the giver of massage should be motivated only by the desire to bestow loving kindness with total concern for the recipient's physical and emotional pains and feelings. Massage given with these motives foremost is a healing experience for the giver as well as the receiver, and intrinsic life energy will flow between the two.

THAI BODYWORK TREATMENT

In order to give and to receive Thai bodywork, you will need a partner – your spouse, friend or perhaps a family member. It's very important that you avoid working with anyone who is much heavier than yourself, particularly when carrying out exercises that may involve heavy lifting or standing on your partner. Thai bodywork is, above all else, an intimate and warm experience and it should be carried out in an environment that promotes these features. A warm, well-ventilated room with diffused or subdued lighting is most conducive to the meditative state of the giver and the relaxation of the receiver. It's important to have no disturbances or excessive noise, although some people may prefer to have gentle background music played throughout the massage. As the bodywork is carried out on the floor, a soft but supportive mat or blanket should be used, together with a thin pillow to support the receiver's head. Adequate space should be provided to enable the giver to move comfortably around the receiver.

Thai massage is applied to the clothed body, although the receiver is usually barefoot. Ideal clothing for both the receiver and the giver, who is also barefoot, is a thin, natural-fibre tracksuit or similar type of loose garment.

Before giving a massage to someone for the first time, it's very important to check their medical history and discuss any present health problems with them (see page 17). Immediately before any physical contact is made, you should take a moment to clear your mind of all extraneous thoughts so as to be totally centred on your partner's needs and to be able to attend to them in a calm and empathetic state. A few slow, deep breaths with controlled exhalation will help this relaxation process.

Before starting a massage, a Thai practitioner says a prayer to the Father of Medicine asking for guidance and help in relieving the physical and emotional pain in the patient. You too can say a prayer if you want.

Throughout the massage your partner should breathe normally except when receiving the 'cobras' (see pages 131-33 and 135) and lifting spinal twist (see page 121). Breathing in deeply before the lifts begin and breathing out as the lifts take place encourages energy flow to the internal organs. As with all forms of massage, pace, rhythm and pressure must be carefully controlled, and, above all else, there must be a sense of continuous flow, not only from technique to technique but also of energies within the partnership between giver and receiver. Wherever possible, the first word used in the headings for the exercises refers to the action of the giver or, where appropriate, the body part used by the giver.

THE DURATION OF A MASSAGE

A Thai massage can take between two and two-and-a-half hours to complete, but this does not preclude the possibility of effective massage when there's less time. It's much better to restrict massage to those regions of the body that can

be adequately treated in the time available than to speed up and try to do a whole body massage in a much shorter time. A selection of short programmes to treat specific conditions is listed in chapter 4. In addition, a basic routine for the beginner appears at the end of the book (see page 154). If you're new to bodywork, don't try the more advanced manipulations until you're able to do the basic routine smoothly and effectively.

BEWARE OF OVERSTRETCHING

Overstretching can cause injury. After just a short experience of giving massage it soon becomes clear that each person has a different pain threshold, sensitivity and overall flexibility. Deep pressure, when applied to some people, produces little more than a mild sensation, whereas for others mild pressure can be quite excruciating. Flexibility and tolerance of stretching show the same variability. It's important to learn to recognize quickly to what degree pressure and stretching can be used. Pressing can cause pain if applied too vigorously, so always start with light pressure and increase slowly. Use visual clues from your partner to guide you as to the maximum pressure.

It's always important to get verbal confirmation from your partner that the stretches are not excessive. Age is no indication of suppleness and pain threshold. Some very young people can be stiff whereas others in their seventies who have looked after their bodies can demonstrate a remarkable flexibility.

CARING FOR YOURSELF

Good balance and posture are vital for the giver of Thai bodywork, as muscular strain can be sustained easily if unnatural and stressful positions are adopted. Leaning in with the full body weight is a far more effective way of applying pressure and performing some of the extensive stretching movements than trying to achieve these with only the muscular power of the arms and shoulders. The giver should feel as comfortable as the receiver, since any discomfort will interrupt concentration and destroy the harmony of movement that's so characteristic of good Thai bodywork.

RHYTHM AND MOVEMENT:
A PURE SYNTHESIS

The words 'flowing' and 'rhythmic' exactly describe the essence of Thai bodywork, with its sequence of unhurried presses, stretches and twists. For the beginner, the vast number, variety and subtlety of techniques used may be somewhat bewildering. At all times, the position and movements of the giver in relation to the receiver are every bit as important as the way in which the techniques are applied. Nuances of tempo and pressure seem endless, and one technique dissolves into another with total smoothness and harmony. Form seems

as important as movement. The symmetries and shapes developed and sustained are as dramatic as the way in which they float away. There is never a suggestion of haste, and to the receiver time seems almost to stand still.

Thai bodywork is a fusion of techniques, each with its own specific effect. Some techniques apply pressure to the Sen lines (see page 12), while others produce the wonderful twists and stretches that often resemble applied yoga. Pressing is the means of stimulating movement of energy in the Sen lines, and manipulations stretch muscles. Feet, palms, thumbs, elbows and knees are the tools of the Thai therapist. The unhurried pace and smooth flow that characterize this form of bodywork also detract from the very deep pressure and powerful stretches that are used. Thai bodywork is like a beautifully choreographed duet: the basic theme is repeated over and over again, but with subtle variations for each body part that's treated.

CONTRAINDICATIONS TO THAI MASSAGE

A few words of caution must be stated. All those incredible shapes and flowing movements that constitute the manipulative side of Thai massage can be potentially damaging to both giver and receiver. To give a massage of this kind, at even a very modest level, requires great skill, strength and poise, which can only be acquired with correct training. Even a fit young person can be hurt when subjected to stretches and twists that are incorrectly applied or simply overdone. Also, there are the usual contraindications to the use of Thai massage, which are essentially those that would apply to any form of massotherapy.

WHEN NOT TO USE THAI BODYWORK

- Don't massage anyone with a serious heart condition, high blood pressure or cancer.
- Thai massage is unsuitable for those who suffer from brittle bones (osteoporosis).
- Never massage anyone who has an artificial joint, such as a hip or knee replacement.
- Those suffering from skin conditions such as eczema, psoriasis or shingles should not receive massage on the affected areas.
- Many of the exercises in this book are unsuitable for pregnant women, and Thai massage isn't recommended during pregnancy.
- Varicose veins shouldn't be deeply massaged.
- If the receiver has any condition that raises doubts in the mind of the giver as to the suitability of this type of massage, it's always best to err on the side of caution and to refer the person to their doctor, who may be able to determine whether massage is contraindicated.

THE MUSCLES

Ageing is often more to do with how we feel than with the passage of time. Decreasing flexibility, stiffness, tension, aches and pains all contribute to the feeling of getting old.

1

Most chronic pain – even headaches – is associated with the musculoskeletal system and originates from muscles that remain contracted (stay shortened) even in their 'relaxed' state. Muscles are the anatomical targets of the Thai masseur.

Skeletal muscle is contractile tissue. It provides the force (effort) for all voluntary movement. Muscles are attached to bone (or sometimes connective tissue or cartilage) by means of tendons. These are flexible and enormously strong, inelastic structures that arise from the connective tissue that covers the muscles. At their outer ends, tendons fuse with connective tissue that covers the bone or cartilage. Whenever a muscle contracts, it shortens, and this creates a pull that's transmitted through the tendons to bring about movement.

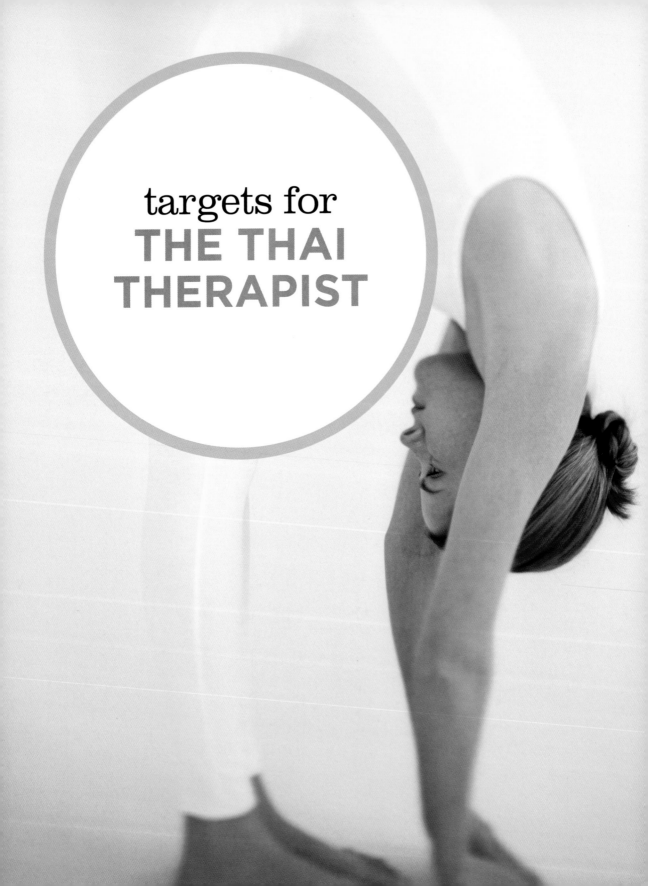

targets for
THE THAI
THERAPIST

THE SUPERFICIAL MUSCLES OF THE BODY

In the living body, the superficial muscles cover layers of deep muscles, which, in turn, may cover even deeper muscles. Seen here, the relationship between the body's natural curves and the superficial muscles beneath the skin and subcutaneous fat is clear. Some deep muscles (shaded orange) can be glimpsed beneath the superficial muscles.

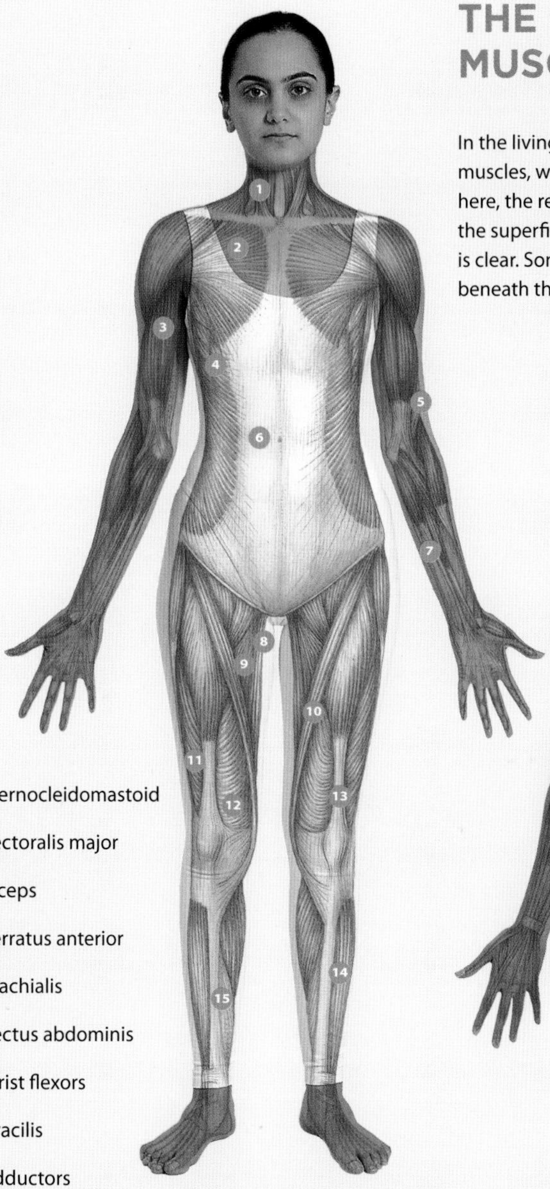

1. Sternocleidomastoid
2. Pectoralis major
3. Biceps
4. Serratus anterior
5. Brachialis
6. Rectus abdominis
7. Wrist flexors
8. Gracilis
9. Adductors
10. Sartorius
11. Vastus lateralis
12. Vastus medialis
13. Rectus femoris
14. Tibialis anterior
15. Soleus

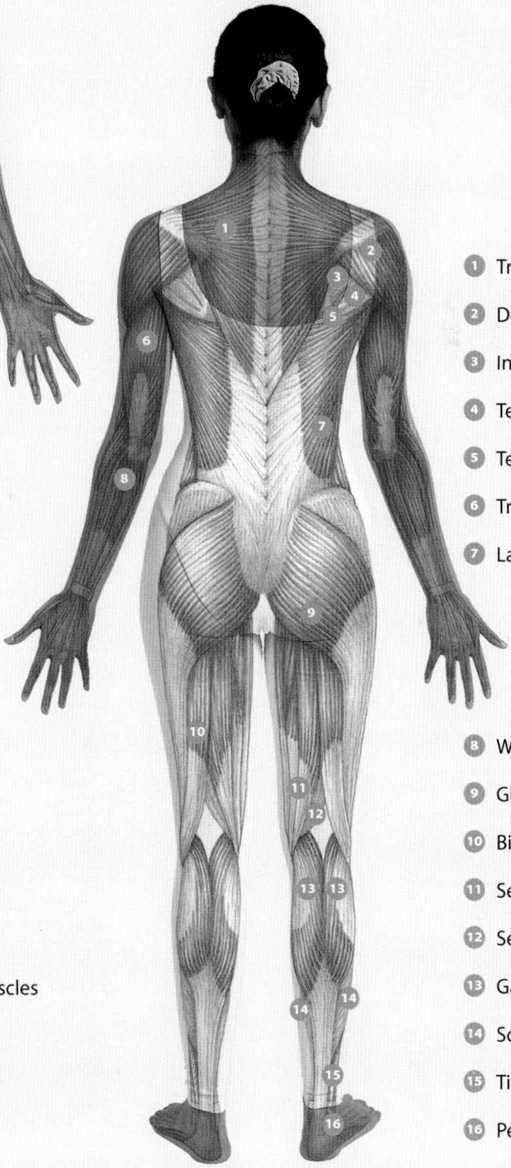

1. Trapezius
2. Deltoid
3. Infraspinatus
4. Teres minor
5. Teres major
6. Triceps
7. Latissimus dorsi
8. Wrist extensors
9. Gluteus maximus
10. Biceps femoris
11. Semitendinosus
12. Semimembranosus
13. Gastrocnemius
14. Soleus
15. Tibialis posterior
16. Peroneus longus

● Superficial muscles
● Deep muscles

HOW MUSCLES WORK

Muscles act on the bones, and these form a very complex system of levers. A muscle is usually attached by its tendons to the bones positioned on either side of a joint. Whenever the muscle contracts, the joint acts like a pivot, and movement is created between the bones.

Muscle cannot work by itself; it depends upon many other tissues, such as myofascia. This not only provides the outer covering for the muscle but also penetrates deep within the muscle, binding together bundles of muscle fibres and carrying nerves and blood capillaries deep into the muscle tissue. Indeed, all the organs of the body depend on connective tissue for support and to bind their various components together. It's connective tissue that forms the supporting framework for the dense network of blood capillaries, nerves and lymph vessels that are essential components of the muscular system. It also provides the ultra-smooth surfaces that enable each muscle to move against its neighbours with almost no friction. Painful adhesions occur when this property of the connective tissue is disturbed.

THE CENTRAL NERVOUS SYSTEM

The brain and spinal cord make up the **central nervous system (CNS)**, which is the controlling computer for all body parts and functions, both voluntary, such as the skeletal muscles, and involuntary, such as breathing. Muscles are linked to the central nervous system by two kinds of nerves:

● **Motor nerves:** these carry nerve impulses from the CNS to make the muscles contract.
● **Sensory nerves:** these carry nerve impulses from sense organs in the muscles to the CNS.

The sense organs in muscles are called **spindle organs** due to their shape. They provide constant information about the state of muscle contraction and any change in it. The tendons also contain sense organs that tell the brain how much pull they are being subjected to as the muscles contract.

WHAT IS A MUSCLE?

A muscle is a bundle of vast numbers of muscle fibres, all arranged lengthwise and parallel with one another. Muscle fibres are the basic contractile

DIAGRAM OF MUSCLE TISSUE (enlarged)

This sectioned muscle shows the arrangement of the tissues that provide for its supporting framework and its contractile ability.

1 Body of muscle

2 Tendon
attaches the muscle to the bone

3 Muscle fascicle
a bundle of muscle fibres

4 Muscle fibre

5 Myofascia
the connective tissue framework of the muscle

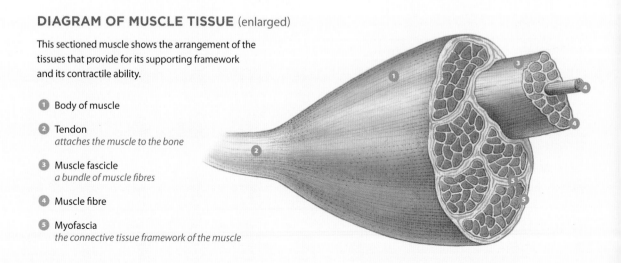

ANTAGONISTIC MUSCLES

Biceps and triceps muscles are the antagonistic pair that provide much of the effort for flexing and extending the arm at the elbow, and raising the arm backwards and forwards at the shoulder.

1. Tendons
2. Scapula
3. Biceps muscle
4. Triceps muscle
5. Humerus
6. Tendons
7. Radius
8. Ulna

FUNCTIONAL MUSCLE GROUPS

Smooth, variable, coordinated movement results from muscles functioning in groups. A group that flexes a joint, for example, interacts with and opposes the action of one that extends it. Two such groups of muscles are said to be **antagonistic**. Biceps and triceps are the main muscles from the antagonistic groups that flex and extend the elbow. Other major functional groups are the quadriceps muscles, which extend the knee and flex the thigh, and the hamstring muscles, which flex the knee and extend the thigh. Each of the four quadriceps and three hamstring muscles work slightly differently from the others to include a degree of rotation in either direction.

MUSCLES AT REST

Muscles can only contract; they can't actively stretch. When a muscle stops contracting, it depends on its antagonists to stretch it back to its normal relaxed length when they contract. Even an apparently relaxed muscle has a small proportion of its fibres in a contracted state. These give a muscle its **tone**. Muscle tone depends on a constant, low-frequency motor-nerve stimulation that originates in the brain. It's just enough to keep the lowest-threshold fibres contracted. Any disturbance of normal tone can seriously affect muscle function. Deficient tone makes the muscle limp and flaccid so that part of its potential contraction is used to 'take up the slack' instead of producing movement. Too much tone deceives the brain into thinking that the muscle is contracting and so inhibits some of the contractile ability of the antagonists, which gradually weaken as a result.

elements within muscles. All muscle fibres have the ability to contract and thus shorten. They contract in an 'all-or-nothing' way – a muscle fibre can't contract just a little. Full contraction or no contraction are the only two possibilities.

Different muscle fibres respond in different ways to the impulses that arrive through motor nerves. Some have what's called 'low threshold response'. This means that they contract under very low frequency of motor-nerve stimulation. Others are far less sensitive and need much higher frequency stimulation. These are said to have a 'high threshold response'. Within the same muscle there are muscle fibres with differing thresholds, to cover the complete spectrum, from low to high. The different response thresholds of the individual muscle fibres allow the muscle to contract smoothly and progressively as more fibres come into action as motor-nerve stimulation increases.

The sheer complexity of muscle interaction is reflected in Thai bodywork, which treats every muscle from every angle.

THE THERAPEUTIC EFFECTS OF THAI BODYWORK

Pressing and stretching are where Thai bodywork excels. At this point it makes sense to look at what happens to our muscles, and how pressing and stretching can help them. One of the most common muscle problems is a gradual shortening of the relaxed muscle length. This has many causes. Those who do too much heavy, repetitive manual work or weight training in the gym can develop muscles with higher than normal tone. This is due to increased numbers of muscle fibres remaining contracted, even when the muscle is in its 'relaxed' state. Other factors such as injury, poor posture and emotional stress can also cause this.

The most immediate effect of muscle shortening is reduced movement at the joint where the muscle works. This is because the difference between the relaxed length and the contracted length of the muscle is less than it should be. It's this difference that determines how much movement the muscle can produce, so stiffness and reduced joint mobility result from muscle shortening.

Other unpleasant conditions can also result. When a muscle becomes tense and shortened, its spindle organs send impulses to the brain, which tell it that the muscle is in a state of contraction. The brain now responds by reducing motor stimulation to its antagonistic muscle, which then loses tone and, if the condition persists, gradually weakens. Soon it will not even match the strength of its antagonist, which will shorten still further since it won't be pulled hard enough to stretch it. Imbalance quickly results, which, in some cases, can produce postural problems leading to chronic pain.

But this isn't the whole story. The myofascia has large areas between its cells that contain fibres – some elastic, some not. The non-elastic ones strengthen the tissue. As a muscle shortens, the myofascia contracts and shortens with it. Gradually it loses some of its elasticity as it's not stretched repeatedly to what should be the correct relaxed length. Non-elastic fibres replace elastic ones, and the tissue becomes slightly wrinkled. Movement of the neighbouring tissues becomes less smooth, causing possible discomfort, which can lead also to abnormal use of the affected parts. As the myofascia shrinks with lack of stretching, it thickens and becomes fibrotic, impeding normal muscle stretching during relaxation and further reducing movement and joint mobility. These interrelated effects mean pain, stiffness, lowered resistance to joint injury and reduced sports performance.

BENEFITS OF PRESSES AND STRETCHES

The deep presses of Thai bodywork squash the muscles, stretching the myofascia sideways. This helps to break down fibrotic tissue and stimulates the production of elastic fibres. Blood flow through the myofascial capillaries is enhanced and energy flow through the Sen is improved. These changes help to alleviate pain and make all the tissues amenable to the effects of stretching.

The large-scale, sustained stretches that characterize Thai manipulations are applied in many different directions. The practitioner constantly changes the angle of approach by altering the relative positions of different parts of the body. Stretching of muscles – even those that are abnormally shortened – takes them just beyond what their normal relaxed length would be. Muscle spindle organs respond to this by 'telling' the brain that the muscle is relaxed; inhibitory nerve impulses to the antagonistic muscles then stop and they soon regain normal tone. Regular Thai bodywork stretches restore balance within and between functional groups of muscles to ease pain, increase flexibility and improve posture.

SHORTENED MUSCLES

The gastrocnemius muscle shown here can be so seriously shortened as a result of wearing high heels that walking barefoot becomes painful. Thai massage easily corrects this condition.

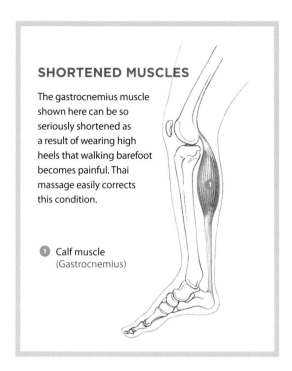

1 Calf muscle
(Gastrocnemius)

KEEPING AND IMPROVING FLEXIBILITY

The overall flexibility of the body's movable joints starts to diminish from the early twenties, unless positive steps are taken to work them through a wide range of movements at regular intervals. You could do this with yoga, but reaching the right level of expertise takes much application and discipline. Thai massage, however, requires nothing more than placing your body in the hands of an expert practitioner. After a session lasting around two to two-and-a-half hours your muscles and joints will have received an intensive workout, more thorough than you could ever achieve on your own. The improvement in your flexibility will be noticeable immediately. This is because Thai bodywork always stretches muscles and manipulates joints just a little further than you could do unaided.

THE TREATMENT OF CONDITIONS

Though unsuitable for people with serious health problems or who have had replacement surgery, for others Thai bodywork can seem miraculous in the way it treats conditions that result from physical and emotional stress. Repetitive strain, sports and wear and tear injuries are the most common results of physical stress. The warning signals vary from stiffness, weakness and pain to serious loss of performance. The indicators of emotional stress are vastly more complex. They can be emotional, such as worry, anxiety and anger, or behavioural, as with overeating and alcohol, tobacco and drug abuse. Inability to relax, disrupted sleep patterns and general irritability can also occur. Eventually, emotional stress leads to a range of physical symptoms, including headaches, indigestion, constipation, back pains and skin conditions.

ENHANCING SPORTS PERFORMANCE

A flexible body is one of the keys to fitness and performance. The other is a musculature with total balance between antagonistic groups, with every individual muscle able to assume its normal relaxed length when not contracting. This is probably a combination that even the most highly trained athletes fail to achieve, although including Thai bodywork as part of a training regime can help every sportsperson reach that goal. It will enable them to undertake more intensive training with a greatly reduced risk of injury, resulting in an ability to sustain even higher levels of performance safely.

TREATING SPORTS INJURIES

Most sports injuries involve damage to muscle fibres, myofascia or tendons, and they are commonly caused by overuse of muscles that are not functionally balanced with other muscles in their group and with their antagonists. A healthy, normal muscle has an amazing capacity to perform repetitively without injury. Regularly received Thai bodywork provides maintenance that the muscles need. When injury does occur, its controlled stretches and manipulations speed healing and restore normal pain-free function.

THE MUSCLES   HEAD & NECK

MUSCLE	REGION/ LESSON	ATTACHMENTS (origin and insertion)	MUSCLE ACTION	KEY THAI MANIPULATIONS ACTING ON THE MUSCLE
ERECTOR SPINAE (Sacrospinalis) (see also page 30)	**Head & neck** lessons 3, 5 & 8	**O:** On all the vertebrae **I:** Upper cervical vertebrae, base of skull and ribs	(Both sides) **Holds neck erect and bends it backwards** (One side) **Flexes head and neck sideways**	• **Bow & arrow spinal twist** (page 89) • **Pulling the turned head** (page 106) • **Interlocked hand/neck press** (page 139) • **Seated lateral arm lever** (page 141) • **Butterfly shoulder stretch** (page 143) • **Butterfly manipulation** (page 143)
STERNOCLEIDO-MASTOID	**Head & neck** lessons 5 & 8	**O:** Mastoid bone behind ear **I:** Top of breast bone (sternum), collarbone (clavicle)	(Both sides) **Tilts head forwards** (One side) **Turns head towards shoulder on that side**	• **Pulling the turned head** (page 106) • **Stretching the neck & shoulders** (page 139) • **Seated lateral arm lever** (page 141)
LEVATOR SCAPULAE	**Head & neck** lessons 3, 5 & 8	**O:** First four cervical vertebrae **I:** Top inner angle of the shoulder blade (scapula)	**Raises shoulder blade and pulls it towards spine**	• **Bow & arrow spinal twist** (page 89) • **Pulling the turned head** (page 106) • **Interlocked hand/neck press** (page 139) • **Seated lateral arm lever** (page 141)
TRAPEZIUS	**Head & neck** lessons 3, 5, 7 & 8	**O:** Base of skull (occiput), cervical vertebrae two to six via the nuchal ligament, and the final cervical and all thoracic vertebrae **I:** Outer end of the collarbone (clavicle), spine of shoulder blade (scapula)	**Rotates and raises shoulder blades** (One side) **Flexes and rotates neck**	• **Bow & arrow spinal twist** (page 89) • **Lifting head to straight knees** (page 95) • **Lifting head to crossed knees** (page 95) • **Foot to armpit stretch** (page 103) • **Pulling the arms** (page 105) • **Pulling the turned head** (page 106) • **Rotating the shoulder** (page 114) • **Lifting spinal twist** (page 121) • **Standing cobra** (page 133) • **Seated lateral arm lever** (page 141)

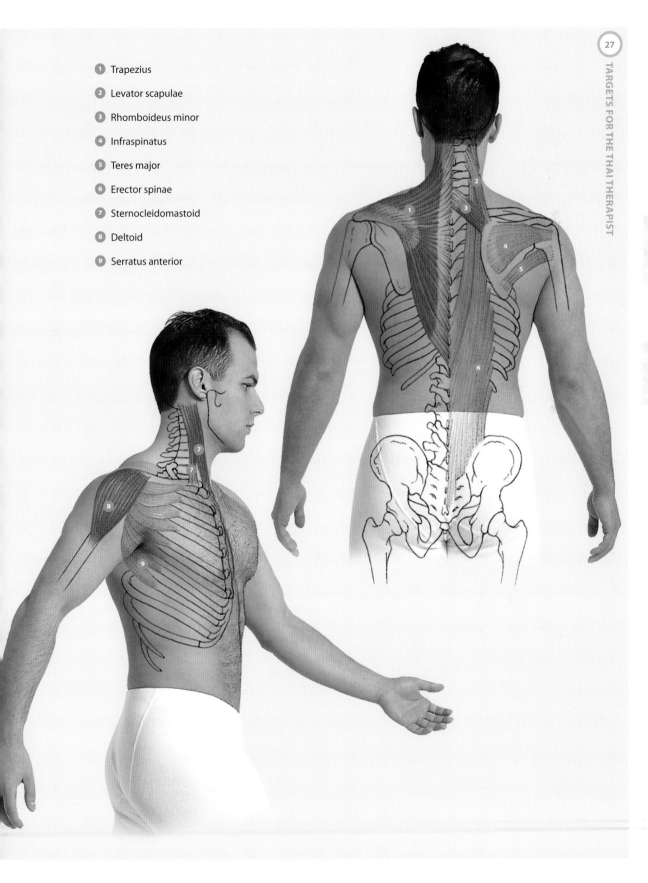

1. Trapezius
2. Levator scapulae
3. Rhomboideus minor
4. Infraspinatus
5. Teres major
6. Erector spinae
7. Sternocleidomastoid
8. Deltoid
9. Serratus anterior

SHOULDERS

MUSCLE	REGION/ LESSON	ATTACHMENTS (origin and insertion)	MUSCLE ACTION	KEY THAI MANIPULATIONS ACTING ON THE MUSCLE
TERES MINOR	**Shoulder** lessons 3, 5 & 8	**O:** Outer margin of shoulder blade (scapula) **I:** Back of the head of humerus	**Rotates arm outwards**	• **Lifting head to straight knees** (page 95) • **Lifting head to crossed knees** (page 95) • **Pulling the arms** (page 105) • **Backwards arm lever** (page 140) • **Elbow pivot lever** (page 140) • **Stretching the arm in the triangle position** (page 103) • **Seated lateral arm lever** (page 141) • **Butterfly shoulder stretch** (page 143)
TERES MAJOR	**Shoulder** lessons 3, 6 & 8	**O:** Lower half of outer margin of shoulder blade (scapula) **I:** Inside margin on upper humerus	**Extends arm backwards and rotates it inwards**	• **Lifting head to straight knees** (page 95) • **Lifting head to crossed knees** (page 95) • **Pulling the arm in the side position** (page 116) • **Stretching the arm in the triangle position** (page 117) • **Backwards arm lever** (page 140) • **Elbow pivot lever** (page 140) • **Seated lateral arm lever** (page 141) • **Butterfly shoulder stretch** (page 143)
SUPRASPINATUS	**Shoulder** lessons 5, 6, 7 & 8	**O:** Shoulder blade above the spine (scapula) **I:** Outer margin on top of humerus	**Raises arm** (abducts)	• **Foot to armpit stretch** (page 103) • **Pulling spinal twist** (page 121) • **Kneeling cushion, sitting stool, standing** and **intimate cobras** (pages 131–33, 135) • **Elbow pivot lever** (page 140) • **Butterfly shoulder stretch** (page 143)
INFRASPINATUS	**Shoulder** lessons 5, 6, 7 & 8	**O:** Inner shoulder blade **I:** Back of head of humerus	**Rotates arm outwards**	as for SUPRASPINATUS (above) • **Rotating the shoulder** (page 114) • **Lifting spinal twist** (page 121)
SUBSCAPULARIS	**Shoulder** lessons 3, 5, 6 & 8	**O:** Front of shoulder blade (scapula) **I:** Inner surface of upper humerus	**Pulls arm downwards, rotates arm towards chest**	as for TERES MINOR (above) • **Lifting spinal twist** (page 121)
DELTOID	**Shoulder** lessons 5, 6, 7 & 8	**O:** Collarbone and scapular spine **I:** Humerus	**Raises arm** (abducts)	as for SUPRASPINATUS (above)
SERRATUS ANTERIOR	**Shoulder** lessons 7 & 8	**O:** Ribs 1–9 **I:** Inner margin of shoulder blade (scapula)	**Antagonistic to rhomboideus muscles, helps to stabilize shoulder blade**	• **Kneeling cushion, sitting stool, standing** and **intimate cobras** (pages 131–33, 135) • **Feet to back stretch** (page 144)

CHEST & ABDOMINAL MUSCLES

MUSCLE	REGION/ LESSON	ATTACHMENTS (origin and insertion)	MUSCLE ACTION	KEY THAI MANIPULATIONS ACTING ON THE MUSCLE
PECTORALIS MAJOR	**Abdomen** lessons 5, 6, 7 & 8	**O:** Collarbone, sternum **I:** Collarbone, sternum	**Rotates arm towards chest, adducts arm**	• **Pulling the arms** (page 105) • **Rotating the shoulder** (page 114) • **Shoulder to opposite knee spinal twist** (page 117) • **Side back bow** (page 119) • **Lateral** and **crossed scissor stretches** (pages 120, 134) • **Kneeling cushion, sitting stool** and **standing cobras** (pages 131–33) • **Backwards arm lever** (page 140) • **Stretching the arm in the triangle position** (page 103) • **Elbow pivot lever** (page 140) • **Butterfly shoulder stretch** (page 143) • **Feet to back stretch** (page 144)

1. Subscapularis

2. Pectoralis major

3. Rectus abdominis

MUSCLE	REGION/ LESSON	ATTACHMENTS (origin and insertion)	MUSCLE ACTION	KEY THAI MANIPULATIONS ACTING ON THE MUSCLE
RECTUS ABDOMINIS	**Abdomen** lessons 3, 6, 7 & 8	**O:** Top of pubic bone **I:** Cartilages of ribs 5–7	**Flexes spine forwards**	• **The half bridge** (page 93) • **Side back bow** (page 119) • **Lateral** and **crossed scissor stretches** (pages 120, 134) • **Kneeling cushion, sitting stool** and **standing cobras** (pages 131–33) • **Feet to back stretch** (page 144)

BACK

MUSCLE	REGION/ LESSON	ATTACHMENTS (origin and insertion)	MUSCLE ACTION	KEY THAI MANIPULATIONS ACTING ON THE MUSCLE
ERECTOR SPINAE (Sacrospinalis) (see also page 26)	**Back** lessons 3, 5 & 8	**O:** On all the vertebrae **I:** Upper-cervical vertebrae, base of skull and ribs	(Both sides) **Extends spine backwards** (One Side) **Twists spine and flexes to one side**	• **Chest to foot thigh pressing** (page 73) • **Praying mantis** (page 74) • **Rotating the hips** (page 89) • **Rocking & rolling the back** (page 90) • **The plough** (page 91) • **Kneeing the buttocks** (page 92) • **Shinning the thighs** (page 93) • **The half bridge** (page 93) • **Lifting head to straight knees** (page 95) • **Lifting head to crossed knees** (page 95) • **Lifting spinal twist** (page 121) • **Pressing head to knees** (page 142) • **Butterfly manipulation** (page 143)
LATISSIMUS DORSI	**Back** lessons 3, 6 & 8	**O:** Lower six thoracic vertebrae, lumbar vertebrae, iliac crests **I:** Front of humerus	**Rotates arm towards chest, pulls arm backwards and inwards**	• **Lifting head to straight knees** (page 95) • **Lifting head to crossed knees** (page 95) • **Stretching the arm in the triangle position** (supine and side) (pages 103, 117) • **Pulling the arm in the side position** (page 116) • **Backwards arm lever** (page 140) • **Elbow pivot lever** (page 140) • **Seated lateral arm lever** (page 141) • **Butterfly shoulder stretch** (page 143)
RHOMBOIDEUS MINOR AND MAJOR	**Back** lessons 5, 6, 7 & 8	**O:** Last cervical and first five thoracic vertebrae **I:** Inner margin of shoulder blade (scapula)	**Pulls shoulder blades** (scapula) **towards spine**	• **Bow & arrow spinal twist** (page 89) • **Lifting head to straight knees** (page 95) • **Lifting head to crossed knees** (page 95) • **Foot to armpit stretch** (page 103) • **Rotating the shoulder** (page 114) • **Lifting spinal twist** (page 121)
QUADRATUS LUMBORUM	**Back** lessons 5, 6, 7 & 8	**O:** Top of iliac crests **I:** Lumbar vertebrae and rib 12	**Sideways bending of lower back**	• **Bow & arrow spinal twist** (page 89) • **Stretching the arm in the triangle position** (page 117) • **Lifting spinal twist** (page 121) • **Knee or hand to buttock/back leg lift** (page 128) • **Seated lateral arm lever** (page 141)

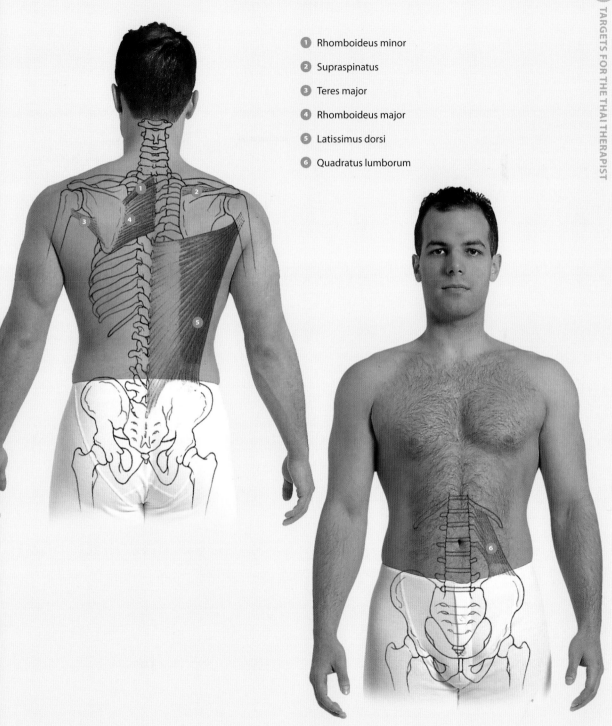

1. Rhomboideus minor
2. Supraspinatus
3. Teres major
4. Rhomboideus major
5. Latissimus dorsi
6. Quadratus lumborum

HIP & BUTTOCK

MUSCLE	REGION/ LESSON	ATTACHMENTS (origin and insertion)	MUSCLE ACTION	KEY THAI MANIPULATIONS ACTING ON THE MUSCLE
GLUTEUS MAXIMUS	Buttocks lessons 2, 3 & 6	O: Sacroiliac joint, back edge of ilium I: Below the head of femur on its posterior surface	Draws leg backwards and rotates thigh outwards	• Chest to foot thigh pressing (page 73) • Praying mantis (page 74) • Rotating the hip (page 75) • The plough (page 91) • Kneeing the backs of the thighs (page 92) • Kneeing the buttocks (page 92) • Shinning the thighs (page 93) • Lifting head to crossed knees (page 95) • Shoulder to opposite knee spinal twist (page 117)

1 Gluteus maximus

2 Piriformis

| PIRIFORMIS | Hips lessons 2 & 6 | O: Front surface of the sacrum
I: Top of femur (great trochanter) | Draws thigh outwards, rotates thigh outwards | • Praying mantis (page 74)
• Rocking the hip (page 79)
• Shoulder to opposite knee spinal twist (page 79)
• Stretching the crossed leg horizontally (pages 80, 118) |

ARMS & HANDS

MUSCLE	REGION/ LESSON	ATTACHMENTS (origin and insertion)	MUSCLE ACTION	KEY THAI MANIPULATIONS ACTING ON THE MUSCLE
BICEPS	Arm lessons 5, 6, 7 & 8	**O:** Scapula (two heads) **I:** Radius	**Flexes arm at elbow**	• **Lifting head to straight knees** (page 95) • **Pulling the arms** (page 105) • **Feet to back stretch** (page 144)
TRICEPS	Arm lessons 5, 6, 7 & 8	**O:** Humerus (two heads), scapula **I:** Ulna	**Extends arm at elbow**	• **Stretching the arm in the triangle position** (supine and side) (pages 103, 117) • **Backwards arm lever** (page 140) • **Elbow pivot lever** (page 140) • **Butterfly shoulder stretch** (page 143)
WRIST & HAND EXTENSORS	Arm lessons 5, 6, 7 & 8	**O:** Humerus, radius, ulna **I:** Wrist bones, hand bones, finger and thumb bones	**Extend palms of hands backwards at wrist, and all the fingers and thumbs**	• **Rotating the wrist** (page 105)
WRIST & HAND FLEXORS	Arm lessons 5, 6, 7 & 8	**O:** Humerus, radius, ulna **I:** Wrist bones, hand bones, finger and thumb bones	**Flex palms of hands upwards at wrist, and fingers and thumbs**	• **Stretching the arm in the triangle position** (supine and side) (pages 103, 117) • **Knee to hand pressing** (page 104) • **Rotating the wrist** (page 105)

1 Biceps
2 Flexors
3 Triceps
4 Extensors

LEGS

MUSCLE	REGION/ LESSON	ATTACHMENTS (origin and insertion)	MUSCLE ACTION	KEY THAI MANIPULATIONS ACTING ON THE MUSCLE
PSOAS MAJOR	**Legs** lessons 6 & 7	**O:** Transverse processes of all lumbar vertebrae and final thoracic vertebra **I:** Femur just below hip joint (lesser trochanter)	**Femur just below hip joint** (lesser trochanter)	• **Swinging the legs** (page 90) • **Knee pivot hip stretch** (page 119) • **Side back bow** (page 119) • **Reverse half lotus leg lift** (page 127) • **Knee or hand to buttock/back leg lift** (page 128) • **Backwards seesaw leg lift** (page 129) • **Standing backwards leg lift** (page 126) • **Kneeling cushion, sitting stool, standing** and **intimate cobras** (pages 131–33, 135) • **Lateral** and **crossed scissor stretches** (page 120) • **Side** and **prone positions** (pages 110, 135) • **Wheelbarrow** (page 134) • **Knee to calf press** (page 135)
ILIACUS	**Legs** lessons 6 & 7	**O:** Front of iliac bones **I:** Together with psoas major	**Flexes thigh up towards abdomen**	as for PSOAS MAJOR (above)
HAMSTRINGS: **BICEPS FEMORIS** **SEMITENDINOSUS** **SEMIMEMBRANOSUS**	**Legs** lessons 2, 3 & 6	**O:** (Biceps femoris) Ischium and posterior upper shaft of femur; (semitendinosus and semimembranosus) ischium **I:** (Biceps femoris) Head of fibula; (semitendinosus) inner surface of tibial shaft; (semimembranosus) inner condyle of the tibia	**Flexes knee, raises lower leg, extends the thigh backwards**	• **Chest to foot thigh pressing** (page 73) • **Praying mantis** (page 74) • **Tug of war** (page 78) • **Pressing in the splits position** (page 80) • **Half lotus back rock & roll** (page 82) • **Vertical half lotus thigh press** (page 83) • **Raised foot leg stretch** (page 84) • **Vertical leg stretch** (page 84) • **The plough** (page 91) • **Lifting head to straight knees** (page 95) • **Knee to knee hip flex** (page 118) • **Stretching the crossed leg horizontally** (page 118)
GRACILIS	**Legs** lessons 2 & 6	**O:** Lower margin of pubic bone **I:** Inner surface of tibial shaft	**Flexes knee, rotates knee inwards, adducts thigh**	• **Tug of war** (page 78) • **Pressing in the splits position** (page 80) • **Half lotus press** (page 81) • **Half lotus back rock & roll** (page 82) • **Corkscrew** (bent leg) (page 83) • **Swinging the legs** (page 90) • **Grape presses** (pages 111–12) • **Knee pivot hip stretch** (page 119) • **Knee or hand to buttock/back leg lift** (page 128)

MUSCLE	REGION/ LESSON	ATTACHMENTS (origin and insertion)	MUSCLE ACTION	KEY THAI MANIPULATIONS ACTING ON THE MUSCLE
SARTORIUS	**Legs** lessons 2 & 7	**O:** Front of iliac bone **I:** Inner surface of upper tibia	Flexes thigh, rotates thigh outwards	• **Pressing the turned-in leg** (page 78) • **Lateral** and **crossed scissor stretches** (pages 120, 134) • **Standing backwards leg lift** (page 126) • **Reverse half lotus leg lift** (page 127) • **Knee or hand to buttock/back leg lift** (page 128) • **Backwards seesaw leg lift** (page 129) • **Wheelbarrow** (page 134)

1. Biceps femoris
2. Semitendinosus
3. Semimembranosus
4. Gastrocnemius
5. Soleus
6. Peroneus longus
7. Tibialis posterior
8. Psoas major
9. Iliacus
10. Vastus lateralis
11. Vastus intermedius
12. Adductors
13. Gracilis
14. Rectus femoris
15. Sartorius
16. Vastus medialis
17. Tibialis anterior

LEGS

MUSCLE	REGION/ LESSON	ATTACHMENTS (origin and insertion)	MUSCLE ACTION	KEY THAI MANIPULATIONS ACTING ON THE MUSCLE
QUADRICEPS: RECTUS FEMORIS VASTUS MEDIALIS VASTUS INTERMEDIUS VASTUS LATERALIS	Legs lessons 2, 3, 6 & 7	(RF) O: Lower iliac spine (Vasti) O: femur I: Patellar (kneecap) ligament to tibia	Extends leg at knee, flexes thigh at hip	• Praying mantis (page 74) • Pressing the turned-in leg (page 78) • Corkscrew (page 83) • The half bridge (page 93) • Pressing the back of the extended leg (page 110) • Pressing the flexed leg (page 110) • Shoulder to opposite knee spinal twist (page 117) • Knee pivot hip stretch (page 119) • Side back bow (page 119) • Foot cracker (page 125) • Pressing feet to buttock (page 126) • Standing backwards leg lift (page 126) • Reverse half lotus leg flex (page 127) • Reverse half lotus leg lift (page 127) • Knee or hand to buttock/back leg lift (page 128) • Backwards seesaw leg lift (page 129) • Wheelbarrow (page 134) • Lateral and crossed scissor stretches (pages 120, 134) • Knee to calf press (page 135)
SOLEUS	Legs lessons 1, 2, 3, 6 & 7	O: Back of upper tibia and fibula I: Heel bone (calcaneus)	Extends foot downwards	AS FOR GASTROCNEMIUS (opposite) • Pressing the feet backwards & forwards (page 58) • Flexing the ankle backwards (page 59)

1 Biceps femoris

2 Peroneus longus

LEGS

MUSCLE	REGION/ LESSON	ATTACHMENTS (origin and insertion)	MUSCLE ACTION	KEY THAI MANIPULATIONS ACTING ON THE MUSCLE
ADDUCTORS	Legs lessons 2, 3 & 6	**O:** Pubic bone and ischium **I:** Inner margin of upper femur	**Draws leg towards midline (adduction)**	• **Pressing the leg in the tree position** (page 68) • **Half lotus press** (page 81) • **Half lotus back rock & roll** (page 82) • **Corkscrew** (page 83) • **Pressing in the splits position** (page 80) • **Swinging the legs** (page 90) • **The plough** (page 91) • **Lifting head to crossed knees** (page 95) • **Grape presses** (pages 111–12) • **Knee pivot hip stretch** (page 119) • **Lateral** and **crossed scissor stretches** (page 120)
PERONEUS LONGUS	Legs lesson 1	**O:** Upper, outer surface of fibula **I:** Base of first metatarsal	**Flexes foot downwards and turns it outwards (everts)**	• **Pressing the feet sideways** (page 56) • **Pressing the crossed feet** (page 57) • **Pressing the feet backwards & forwards** (page 58)
TIBIALIS ANTERIOR	Legs lessons 1 & 7	**O:** Outer margin of tibia **I:** Base of metatarsal bones	**Flexes foot upwards at ankle and turns it inwards**	• **Pressing feet & ankles** (page 56) • **Pressing the feet sideways** (page 56) • **Pressing the feet backwards & forwards** (page 58) • **Pressing the crossed feet** (page 57) • **Stretching the arched foot** (page 62) • **Pressing thigh to calf** (page 76) • **Pressing heel to buttock** (page 125) • **Pressing the thigh & pulling the foot** (page 125) • **Foot cracker** (page 125) • **Reverse half lotus leg flex** (page 127)
TIBIALIS POSTERIOR	Legs lessons 1	**O:** Posterior of tibia and fibula upper shafts **I:** Third and fourth metatarsals	**Flexes foot arch, turns foot inwards and supports the arch**	• **Pressing the feet sideways** (page 56) • **Pressing the feet backwards & forwards** (page 58) • **Flexing the ankle backwards** (page 59)
GASTROCNEMIUS	Legs lessons 2, 3, 6 & 7	**O:** Inner surface and outer surface of lower femur **I:** Heel bone (calcaneus) via the Achilles tendon	**Extends foot downwards and flexes leg at knee**	• **Flexing & stretching the leg** (page 77) • **Pressing in the splits position** (page 80) • **Rocking & rolling the back** (page 90) • **Lifting head to straight knees** (page 95) • **Vertical leg stretch** (page 84) • **Stretching the crossed leg horizontally** (pages 80, 118) • **Knee to calf press** (page 135)

KEY ACUPRESSURE POINTS

The acupressure points in this book have been carefully chosen by Maria Mercati because they can be easily assimilated into a Thai massage routine and individually have powerful therapeutic effects that will totally transform your Thai massage. Each acupressure point needs firm, repetitive kneading to produce its effect.

	ANATOMICAL LOCATION	FUNCTION
FOOT		
K 1	On the midline of the sole, two-thirds along from the back of the heel	• **Restores consciousness** • **Calms the mind for good sleep**
K 3	Midway between the tip of the inner ankle bone and the Achilles tendon	• **Strengthens and treats the lumbar spine and knees** • **Promotes restful sleep**
K 5	One thumb width below K 3	• **Local point for heel and ankle pain**
K 6	Directly below the inner ankle bone	• **Treats lower back pain and insomnia**
BL 64	Opposite SP 4 on the lateral side of the foot on the proximal end of fifth metatarsal	• **Treats neck and lower back stiffness and pain**
SP 4	In the centre of the arch of the foot on the proximal end of first metatarsal	• **Regulates spleen and stomach functions**
ST 41	In the middle of the crease on the front of the ankle	• **Strengthens the ankle and treats ankle pain** • **Treats frontal headache**
LIV 3	In the groove between the first and second toes	• **Calms emotions, reduces stress and treats migraines and PMT**
GB 40	At lower front edge of the outer ankle bone	• **Strengthens the ankle and treats ankle pain**
FRONT & SIDE LEG		
SP 9	Slide up the inside edge of the tibia to the knee to where bone flares – opposite GB 34	• **Prevents and reduces swollen legs** • **Relieves local pain and knee pain**
SP 6	Under the inside edge of the tibia, four finger widths above the inner ankle bone **Contraindicated when pregnant**	• **Improves digestion** • **Prevents and reduces swollen legs** • **Regulates menstruation**
ST 36	Four finger widths below the lateral knee eye and one thumb width from the crest of the tibia	• **Boosts the immune system and promotes health and longevity** • **Lowers high blood pressure** • **Aids digestion and eases gastrointestinal discomfort**
GB 34	In a depression, just in front of and below the head of the fibula	• **Relaxes tendons for the whole body** • **Treats muscle spasm in the leg**
ST 31	On the thigh on a line from the lateral kneecap to the iliac crest, level with the pubic bone	• **Treats pain in the hip joint** • **Treats lower back pain and leg pain in the rectus femoris muscle**

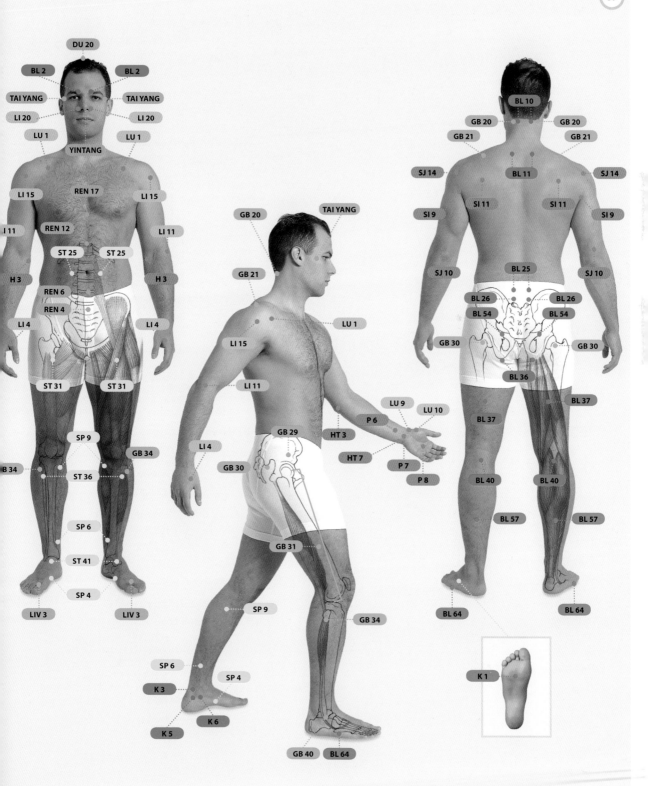

KEY ACUPRESSURE POINTS

	ANATOMICAL LOCATION	FUNCTION
ABDOMEN		
REN 12	On the midline, midway between navel and sternum tip	• **Strengthens the stomach for better digestion** (page 98)
REN 4	Approximately three finger widths above the centre of the pubic bone	• **Strengthens the kidneys to improve vitality and fertility** • **Regulates menstruation**
REN 6	Two finger widths below the navel	• **Energizes the body**
ST 25	Approximately three finger widths lateral to the centre of the naval	• **Improves bowel function** • **Treats abdominal pain and bloating**
CHEST		
LU 1	Under the lateral end of the clavicle, between the first and second ribs	• **Strengthens the lungs to prevent colds, relieves coughs, sore throats and asthma**
REN 17	On midline of breast bone level with the nipples	• **Promotes blood circulation in the heart** • **Eases chest congestion and restores a sense of calm**
HAND		
LI 4	In the V-shaped fleshy area between thumb and forefinger **Contraindicated when pregnant**	• **Strengthens the immune system. Eases pain anywhere in the body. Relieves headaches, toothache, runny and blocked nose**
P 6	Three finger widths above the inside wrist crease on the midline between the two tendons	• **Relieves nausea and motion sickness** • **Important point for preventing cardiovascular problems**
P 7	On the middle of the inside wrist crease	• **Treats carpal tunnel pain and palpitations, and calms**
P 8	Where the third finger touches the palm	• **Restores spiritual and emotional balance**
HT 7	Next to P 7 on the little finger side	• **Treats sleeping disorders caused by emotional issues**
LU 9	Next to P 7 on the thumb side	• **Strengthens lung energies to prevent colds**
LU 10	In the middle of the fleshy pad at the base of the thumb	• **Relieves arthritis in the thumb joint** • **Soothes a sore, swollen throat**
ELBOW		
HT 3	At medial end of elbow crease	• **Relieves pain of golfer's elbow and benefits heart function**
LI 11	At the outer end of the elbow crease	• **Relieves pain of tennis elbow and lowers high blood pressure**
SJ 10	In a depression, about two finger widths above the base of the humerus	• **Treats elbow and triceps muscle pain**
SHOULDER/ARM		
LI 15	On the anterior deltoid about two finger widths below the front of the corner of the acromion	• **Boosts energy flow in the shoulder to improve mobility and ease pain**
SJ 14	On the posterior deltoid about two finger widths below the corner of the acromion	
SI 9	One thumb width above the back of the armpit	
SI 11	In the centre of the scapula on infraspinatus	

	ANATOMICAL LOCATION	FUNCTION

FACE & HEAD

YINTANG	Midway between the eyebrows	• **Calms the mind and promotes restful sleep**
DU 20	On the midline top of the head, laterally level with the top of the ears	• **Relaxes the mind and improves memory** • **Relieves headaches**
BL 2	On the inner tips of the eyebrows	• **Improves eye health, treats headaches and clears sinuses**
TAI YANG	In the depression on the temples	• **Calms restlessness to aid sleep, treats headaches and relieves eye strain**
LI 20	On either side of the nostrils	• **Clears the nasal passages and stops a runny nose**

HIP IN SIDE POSITION

GB 30	One-third of the distance along a line drawn from the outer edge of the hip bone to the coccyx	• **Improves energy flow through the hip to treat sciatica, hip joint, buttock and lower leg pain**
GB 29	On the side, halfway between the top front of the iliac crest and the hip bone	• **Treats side hip and side leg pain**
GB 31	On the side of the thigh, just less than halfway from the knee crease to the hip bone	• **Treats side leg pain and sciatica** • **Soothes itching**

BACK & LEGS

BL 11 ↓ BL 26	Bladder points from cervical 7 (C 7) to lumbar 5 (L 5) vertebrae, located two finger widths from the centre of the spine	• **Each point represents one of the major organs and should be pressed to powerfully balance all vital processes**
BL 25 BL 26	Level with the tip of the spinous processes of lumbar vertebrae 4 and 5	• **Maintains healthy lower back and treats backache and sciatica**
BL 54	Four finger widths, level with the lower border of the sacrum	
BL 36	Middle of the crease below the buttock	• **Treats painful hamstring muscles, lumbar and sciatic pain**
BL 37	Approximately halfway between BL 36 and knee crease	
BL 40	At the midpoint of the knee crease	• **Reduces knee and back stiffness and pain**
BL 57	Halfway between BL 40 and the ankle	• **Relieves lower back and calf muscle pain**

NECK & SHOULDERS

GB 20	At the top of the nape of the neck in a depression, below the base of the skull	• **Relaxes tendons in the neck to ease tension headaches and neck pain. Prevents and relieves high blood pressure**
GB 21	Halfway between the centre of the spine and the outer edge of the acromium	• **Tension-relief point for pain and stiffness in the shoulder and neck**
BL 10	To the side of the midline below base of the neck	• **Relieves central neck pain**

THE MECHANICS OF THAI MASSAGE

• • • • • • • • • • • • • • • • • •

To create the fundamental effect of pressure that is necessary for Thai bodywork, force is applied by the masseur. 'Soft tissue massage' and 'manipulation' describe the two key techniques of Thai bodywork.

In soft tissue massage, pressure is used directly to reach the desired effect. For the manipulative techniques, pressure is used to achieve stretching and twisting. Traditional Thai bodywork massage is remarkable for the number of different positions in which the receiver's body is presented to the masseur, who also has to adopt a corresponding variety of body positions.

Many of the manipulations in Thai bodywork involve substantial leverage. This often works to the advantage of the practitioner by enabling a small effort to achieve a large effect. This will also benefit the receiver provided that care is taken to avoid overstretching, which could occur if manipulations were performed too quickly.

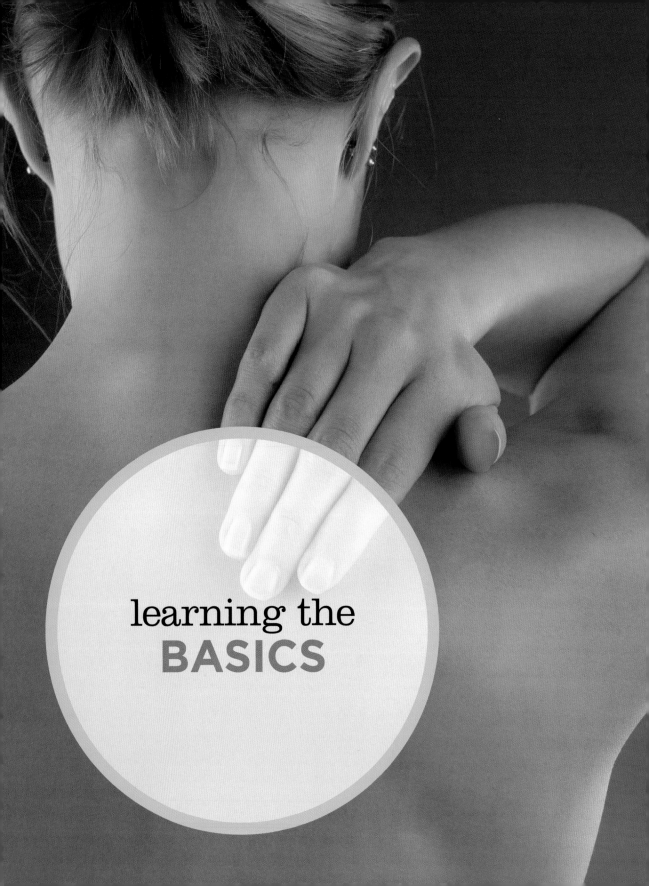

learning the
BASICS

SOFT TISSUE PRESSURE TECHNIQUES

Pressing is the basis of all soft tissue massage techniques. Skilful application of pressure can affect different levels within the tissues and enhances the flow of energy. The application of a force through a larger body surface, such as the palm of the hand or the sole of the foot, creates a pressure that's spread out and doesn't penetrate too deeply. If the same force is applied with the thumb or the tip of the elbow to cover a smaller area, a much more focused and penetrating pressure results. For all pressure techniques, always start with light pressing and increase gradually. Some people find very deep pressure extremely painful.

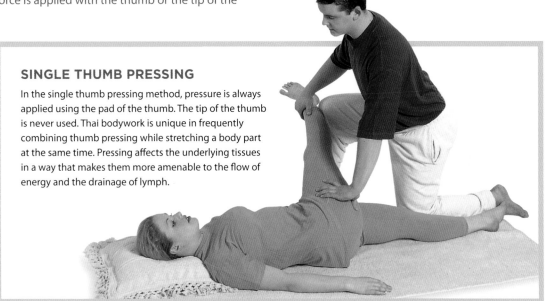

SINGLE THUMB PRESSING

In the single thumb pressing method, pressure is always applied using the pad of the thumb. The tip of the thumb is never used. Thai bodywork is unique in frequently combining thumb pressing while stretching a body part at the same time. Pressing affects the underlying tissues in a way that makes them more amenable to the flow of energy and the drainage of lymph.

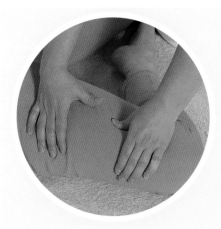

THUMB WALKING

This method is used to stimulate the energy pathways (see page 12). Movement can be in either direction along the lines. The thumbs are placed with their tips almost touching and pressed alternately as they progress along the energy pathways. If movement is towards the left, the left thumb is lifted and moved two to three centimetres (three-quarters to one inch) to the left, and pressure is applied. The right thumb is then moved up to join the left and pressed in turn.

This sequence is repeated over and over again so that alternate thumb pressure is applied along the whole length of the energy pathways. The thumb 'walking' can also be done from left to right.

PALM PRESSING

The palmar surface of the hand is extensively used for applying strong pressure over larger areas of the body than would be possible with the thumbs. Pressure can be applied and sustained without movement, either for a few seconds or up to several minutes. Palmar pressing can be used to create a rocking action, which is achieved with short-duration presses. The upper body weight over the arms is used to generate strong and sustained pressure. To reach the effect required without fatigue, the arms are usually kept straight. There are three different ways of pressing with the palmar surface – single palm pressing, double palm pressing and butterfly palm pressing.

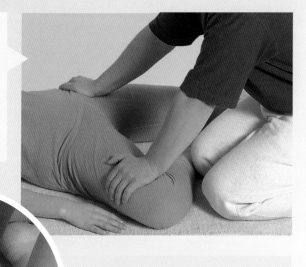

SINGLE PALM PRESSING
The emphasis here is often on the heel of the hand, and the technique is used for applying firm pressure to the major soft tissue masses of the body, such as the back, buttocks and thighs.

CAUTION
For all pressure techniques, start with light pressing and gradually increase.

DOUBLE PALM PRESSING
Here, concentration of the pressure is achieved by placing one hand directly on top of the other.

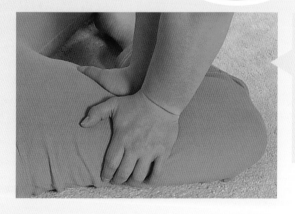

BUTTERFLY PALM PRESSING
This method involves simultaneous pressure using both hands, with the heels of the palms touching. It spreads the force over an even wider area of the body.

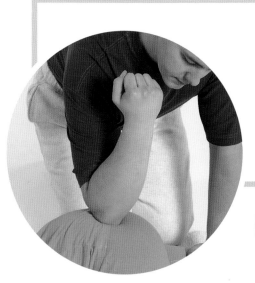

ELBOW PRESSING

Using elbow pressing with the tip of the elbow, the masseur can apply deeper pressure than is possible with the hand. It's used on the thighs, buttocks and upper shoulders, where the muscles are thick. If the elbow tip causes too much pain, the upper forearm can be used instead to spread the force and to reduce pressure.

CAUTION
For all pressure techniques, start with light pressing and gradually increase.

KNEE PRESSING

Used mainly on the backs of the legs and buttocks, knee pressing frees the hands for controlling stretches, while, at the same time, exerting deep pressure.

FOOT PRESSING

The foot is ideally shaped to apply pressure over large areas of the body. On strongly curved parts, such as thighs, the arch is used, but for thickly muscled buttocks and similar muscular areas, the heel or the front of the sole can create strong, penetrating pressure. For some manipulations, parts of the body are pulled against the foot to give a powerful stretch.

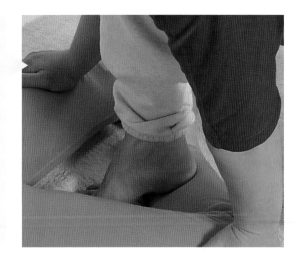

CAUTION

For all pressure techniques, start with light pressing and gradually increase.

BUTTOCK PRESSING

Controlled sitting, where more or less of the weight is taken on the practitioner's feet or knees, is sometimes applied. This is particularly useful as a way to anchor one part of the body

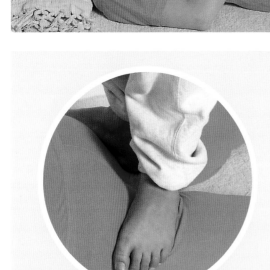

STANDING PRESSURE

Foot pressure from a standing position can be extremely penetrating and should be applied with great care. It's used on the back, buttocks, legs and feet.

THE BENEFITS OF PRESSING

Pressure sense organs in the skin produce pleasurable sensations when subjected to large-scale and sustained pressing. Too much pressure, however, creates discomfort or pain. Concentrated pressure on the energy channels boosts energy flow, and deep pressure on the tissues encourages the release of adhesions in the connective tissue (myofascia) that surrounds the muscles. Blood flow in superficial capillaries and lymphatic drainage is also aided by all kinds of pressing.

MANIPULATION TECHNIQUES

Manipulation is the controlled movement of one or more parts of the body relative to others to achieve specific effects, such as stretching and twisting. It always involves leverage. The masseur must have a high sensitivity to its effectiveness, which can result in very powerful stretches and twists with relatively little effort. A lack of this sensitivity could result in injury. In order to avoid serious back strain caused by lifting and moving in the wrong way, the giver should also be constantly aware of their own posture and position relative to the receiver.

THE BENEFITS OF MANIPULATIONS

Thai manipulations work on the theory that, to be effective, the manipulation must always take the movement just a little further than the recipient would be capable of doing themselves unaided. A good Thai practitioner always knows exactly how far a movement can be taken without causing pain or injury to the recipient. Regular Thai bodywork progressively develops a degree of flexibility and mobility in the body that many recipients find amazing.

With Thai manipulations, there's a complex interaction between giver and receiver. This allows certain parts of the body to be reached that other forms of massage leave untreated.

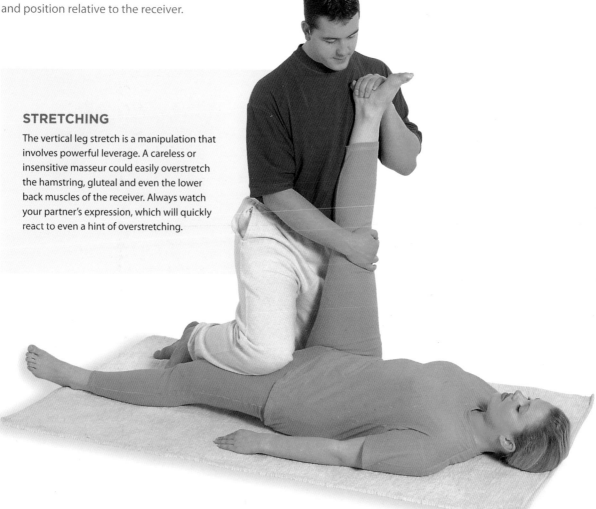

STRETCHING

The vertical leg stretch is a manipulation that involves powerful leverage. A careless or insensitive masseur could easily overstretch the hamstring, gluteal and even the lower back muscles of the receiver. Always watch your partner's expression, which will quickly react to even a hint of overstretching.

PREPARATION FOR MANIPULATION

All the different parts of the body are manipulated during Thai bodywork, and manipulation is achieved through pulling, pushing, lifting, shaking and rotating. The end result of these manipulations are stretching and twisting.

So impressive are the Thai manipulations that the therapist can be tempted to emphasize them at the expense of pressing techniques. This is a serious mistake. Pressure on the soft tissues prepares the receiver physiologically so that the greatest benefit can be derived from the manipulations that follow them. It's the pressure techniques that are most effective in the treatment of pain and in stimulating the flow of energy in the Sen/Meridians.

LIFTING

Most manipulations involve some lifting, which means pulling against the receiver's weight. A lift is a simple manipulation, where the body part is raised against the force of gravity. No pushing is used.

SHAKING

This technique is carried out on the limbs and it always involves an up and down movement. A slight pull creates a degree of traction, which makes the shaking even more effective.

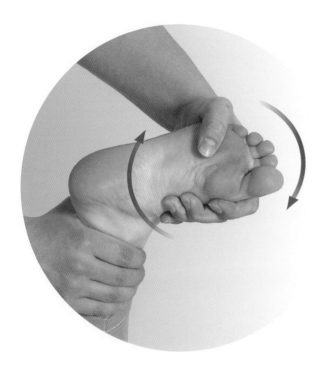

ROTATION

This is a 360° movement of joints such as the wrists, ankles, shoulders, hips and neck. It's the result of alternate pushing and pulling techniques. Even joints affected by osteoarthritis can have normal mobility restored through regular rotation.

PULLING AND PUSHING

Whenever a body part is pulled, it must be anchored at its other end. Sometimes the subject's body weight achieves this. However, the strongest pulling often requires an opposing push. Thai therapists frequently use their feet for this. The most powerful sustained pulls are achieved when the practitioner's body weight is used to generate the effort. Leaning away from the subject creates this effect.

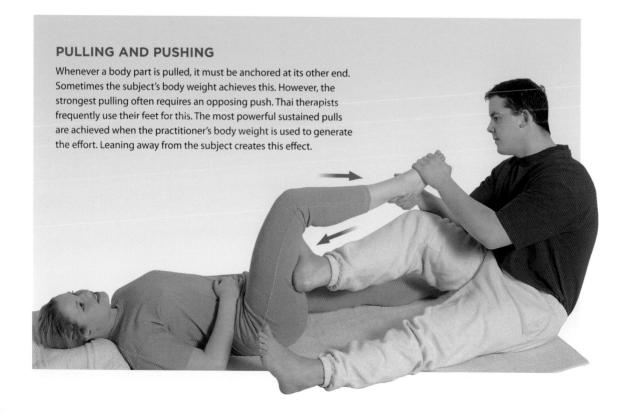

THAI BODYWORK PROGRAMME

· · · · · · · · · · · · · · · · ·

In Thailand there are many subtle variations in both the techniques and the massage sequence. The sequence shown in the following pages presents a unique, whole body programme, devised by Maria Mercati and based on a synthesis of techniques from northern and southern Thailand.

Each step is accompanied by a demonstration photograph. Some photos have arrows or coloured dots superimposed to show you exactly where to apply pressure, and which acupressure points to knead. The healing benefits and key muscles used in each massage are listed alongside. Caution boxes indicate where you should take care with a particular technique, but it should be emphasized here again that Thai massage isn't recommended during pregnancy.

THAI MASSAGE ROUTINE

LESSON	POSITION OF SUBJECT	PARTS OF BODY MASSAGED
ONE	supine (lying on the back)	• both feet simultaneously • each foot individually
TWO	supine	• both feet and legs simultaneously • left leg only • right leg only
THREE	supine	• both legs simultaneously and back
FOUR	supine	• abdomen • chest
FIVE	supine	• arms and hands individually • face, neck, shoulders and head
SIX	lying on the left or right side	• repetition of all parts of the body that can be reached in the side position – NB the left side is a mirror image of the right side
SEVEN	prone (lying face downwards)	• legs • back • arms
EIGHT	sitting	• shoulders and neck • face • head

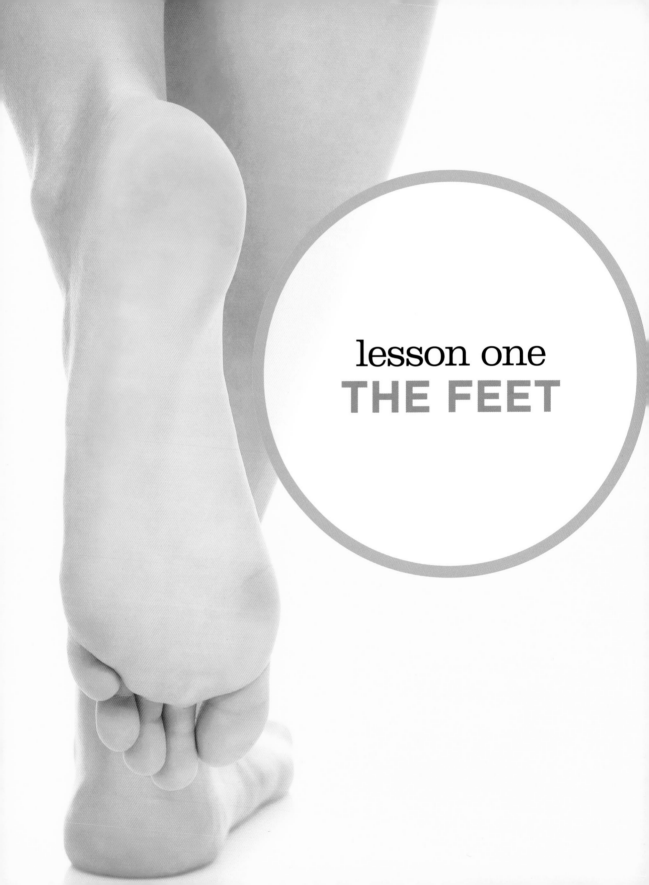

lesson one
THE FEET

The massage starts here. Since this is the first physical contact between the giver and receiver, the scene should be set very carefully (see pages 16–17). To receive massage, your partner should be lying comfortably in the supine position (on the back) with arms in a relaxed position down the sides of the body, and legs apart, leaving a gap of one body-width between the feet. The aim of Lesson One is to stimulate the energy flow through the feet to affect the whole body. See pages 42–51 for the basic techniques of pressing and manipulation.

SEN/MERIDIANS ON THE FEET

The five Thai Sen lines on the soles of the feet all start at a point on the front margin of the heel pad on the midline. They radiate from this point to the toes. K 1 on the Kidney Meridian is halfway along the middle Sen line.

Thumb press from the centre heel point towards each toe, working both feet together. Press the Sen lines as many times as the strength of your thumb allows. Feet bear the weight of the whole body as well as moving to walk and run, so they require both flexibility and strength. Working through the techniques in this lesson will help your partner to maintain foot flexibility and avoid injury.

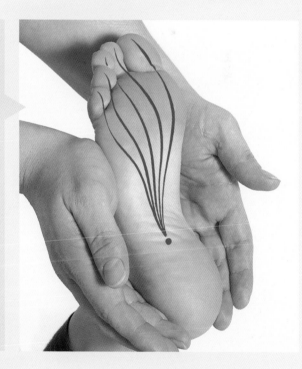

These are the five Sen on the sole of the foot. Thorough pressing of these Sen is regarded as a vital prelude to overall energy balance.

MASSAGING BOTH FEET

HEALING BENEFITS

Warms and loosens the feet
and has a relaxing effect
on the recipient.

Twists the thighs outwards
and exercises the hip.

1 PRESSING FEET & ANKLES

Kneeling between your partner's legs, grasp
both feet. Keep your arms straight so that your
body weight can be transferred through them.
Rock forwards and outwards or from side to side,
increasing pressure through the palms. Move your
palms down the inner margins of your partner's feet
towards the toes, using pressure at each position.

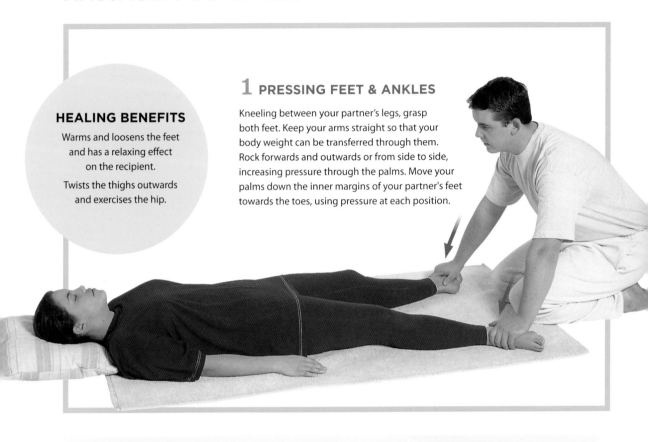

2 PRESSING THE FEET SIDEWAYS

Press your partner's feet outwards (evert) as far as they
will stretch and hold them in place for a few seconds.
Release the feet, place your hands across the top
part of the feet and press them inwards (invert) as
shown, right. Repeat the sequence once or twice.

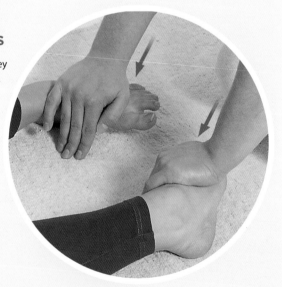

HEALING BENEFITS

Improves ankle
flexibility.

3 PRESSING THE CROSSED FEET

Bring your partner's feet together to cross one foot over the other. Apply gentle, sustained downwards pressure on them, then reverse positions and press again.

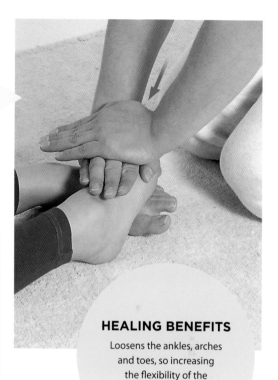

MUSCLES STRETCHED & PRESSED

1 Pressing feet & ankles
Stretched: TIBIALIS ANTERIOR (outwards)

2 Pressing the feet sideways
Stretched: TIBIALIS ANTERIOR (outwards), TIBIALIS POSTERIOR (inwards), PERONEUS LONGUS (inwards)

3 Pressing the crossed feet
Stretched: PERONEUS LONGUS, TIBIALIS POSTERIOR

HEALING BENEFITS

Loosens the ankles, arches and toes, so increasing the flexibility of the tarso-metatarsal joints.

4 SQUEEZING THE FEET

Grasp the tops of your partner's feet, pressing K 3, and squeeze firmly and progressively down towards the toes, pressing SP 4 and BL 64 as you go. Repeat several times.

HEALING BENEFITS

Stimulates the inner and outer foot Sen/Meridians.

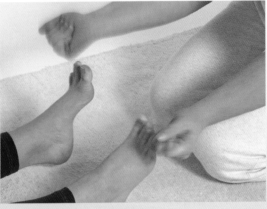

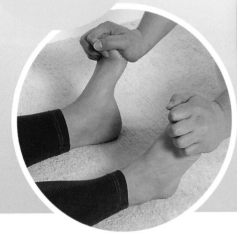

5 FLICKING THE TOES

Place the heel of your hand under your partner's toes and close your fingers above all the toes. Slide your hands off the toes, flicking them upwards as you do so. Then repeat technique 1.

6 PRESSING THE FEET BACKWARDS & FORWARDS

Place the heels of your palms under your partner's toes and firmly push towards the head. Then with your palms on top of the toes, press downwards.

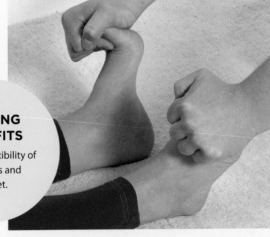

HEALING BENEFITS

Improves flexibility of the ankles and the feet.

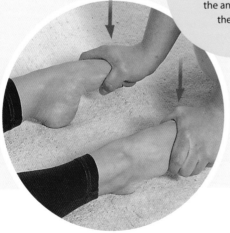

MUSCLES STRETCHED & PRESSED

Pressing the feet backwards & forwards
Stretched: PERONEUS LONGUS (upwards), TIBIALIS POSTERIOR (upwards), SOLEUS (upwards), TIBIALIS ANTERIOR (downwards)

7 PRESSING POINTS ON ANKLES & FEET

Thumb press deeply into the ankle points K 3, K 5 and K 6, marked here with dots. Thumb press the undersides of the heels and then along the energy lines (see page 55) to the toes.

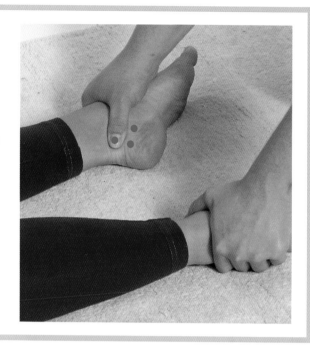

HEALING BENEFITS

K 3, K 5 and K 6 maintain a healthy back and knees.

MASSAGING EACH FOOT INDIVIDUALLY

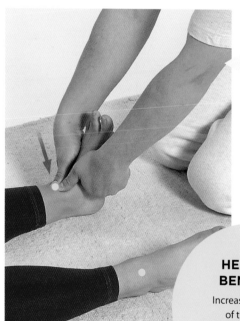

1 FLEXING THE ANKLE BACKWARDS

Grasp your partner's foot with both hands, pressing your thumbs into the centre of the front ankle crease to press ST 41. Then lean forwards to press the foot upwards against this pressure.

MUSCLES STRETCHED & PRESSED

Flexing the ankle backwards
Stretched: PERONEUS LONGUS (upwards), TIBIALIS POSTERIOR (upwards), SOLEUS

HEALING BENEFITS

Increases flexibility of the ankle.

ST 41 refreshes the head and clears headaches.

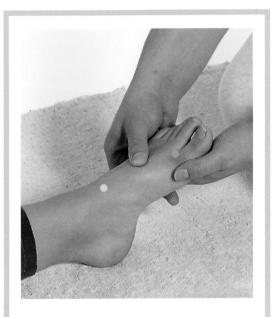

3 PULLING & CRACKING EACH TOE

Hold each of your partner's toes, lean back and pull vigorously in turn. During this technique a cracking sound may be heard.

2 PRESSING THE TENDONS OF THE UPPER FOOT

With circular movements, thumb press the tendons. Begin at ST 41 and work your way towards the toes, following each tendon in turn. Knead LIV 3.

HEALING BENEFITS

Increases blood flow around the tendons, which helps to maintain foot flexibility.

LIV 3 has a calming effect and clears energy blockages in the body.

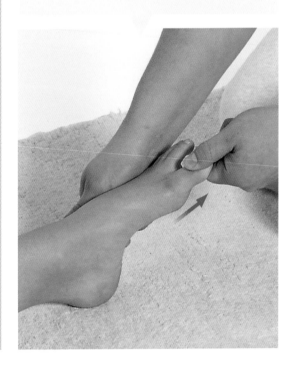

4 TWISTING THE FEET

Support your partner's foot with one hand and bend the free edge of the foot up and down with a twisting, flicking action. Do this two to three times while working towards the toes. Repeat the sequence on the opposite side of the foot.

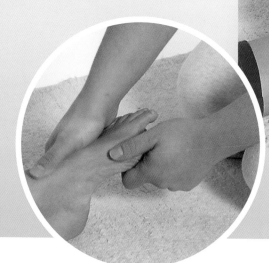

HEALING BENEFITS

Stimulates the foot and increases lateral flexibility.

The intrinsic muscles of the foot are well stretched during the twisting movements.

HEALING BENEFITS

Brings the recipient's awareness into the tips of the toes, which is invigorating.

Start and end points of the Sen/Meridians are massaged to improve overall energy balance.

5 MASSAGING THE TOES

Touch method one: fast toe pulling
Start by rapidly pulling all your partner's toes. Use all your fingers simultaneously and work with a rapid snapping action as the toes are released.

Touch method two: rotating & squeezing
Rotate each of your partner's toes both ways. Follow this with a firm squeezing action towards the tip of the toes and release with a sliding movement.

Touch method three: toe tip massage
Here, the toe is held between two fingers and the extreme tip is massaged vigorously with a circular motion.

6 STRETCHING THE ARCHED FOOT

Grasp your partner's foot with your thumbs over the front of the ankle. Lean back as you press down with the base of your thumbs to stretch the foot into an arched position. Repeat this stretch twice: first, with your hands around the instep and then again nearer the toes, which are arched downwards.

HEALING BENEFITS

Improves flexibility of the foot and opens the knee and hip joints.

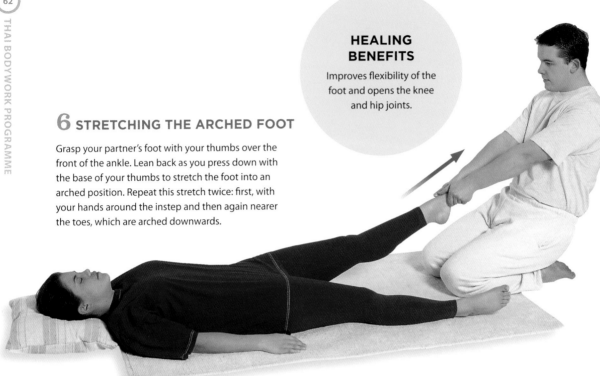

MUSCLES STRETCHED & PRESSED

6 Stretching the arched foot
Stretched: FOOT FLEXORS, TIBIALIS ANTERIOR

7 Rotating the foot
Stretched: SOLEUS, FOOT EXTENSORS and FLEXORS

7 ROTATING THE FOOT

Support your partner's leg above the ankle, firmly grasp the foot, press into GB 40 while rotating it several times in both directions.

HEALING BENEFITS

GB 40 Improves flexibility of the ankles.

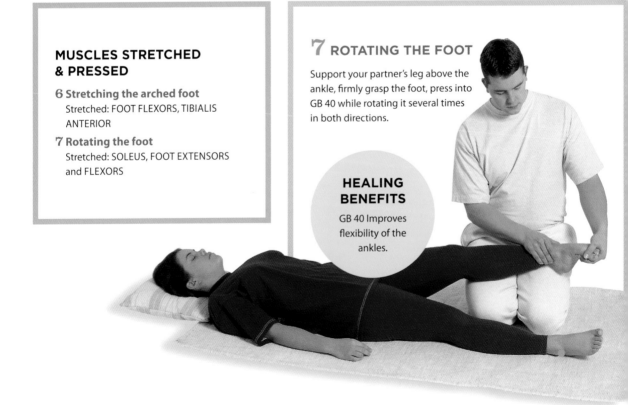

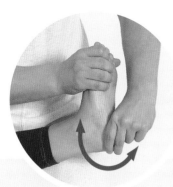

8 ROTATING THE HEEL

Grasp your partner's heel as shown and then rotate it with a simultaneous squeezing action.

HEALING BENEFITS

Creates a feeling of groundedness and vibrates the hip joint.

10 PUMMELLING THE HEEL

Stretching your partner's toes towards the head, pummel the underside of the heel using your clenched fist.

Now repeat techniques 1–10, as described above, on the other foot.

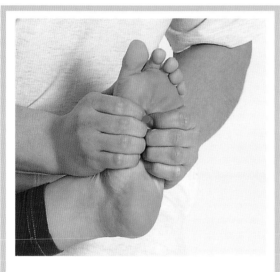

9 PRESSING THE FOOT SEN

Grasp your partner's foot in both hands, dig your fingertips into the sole and press deeply with a squeezing action into the central and then the two lateral Sen lines in turn. Thumb press along all five Sen lines (see page 55). Press and knead K 1 at least 50 times.

HEALING BENEFITS

Improves foot flexibility. K 1 boosts energy flow for well-being.

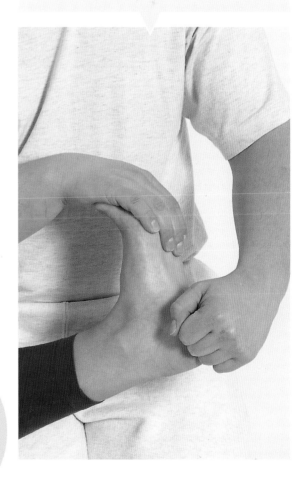

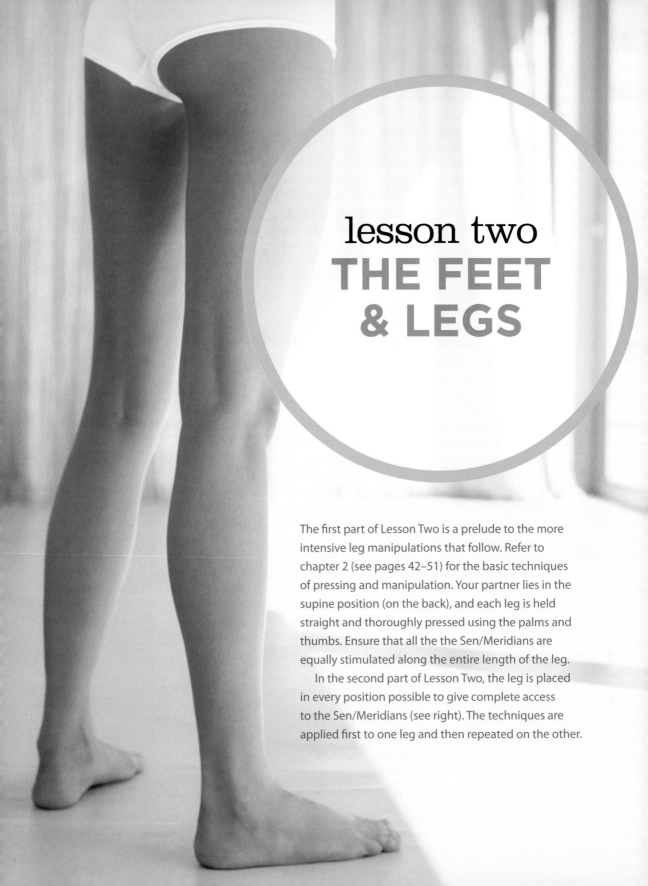

lesson two
THE FEET & LEGS

The first part of Lesson Two is a prelude to the more intensive leg manipulations that follow. Refer to chapter 2 (see pages 42–51) for the basic techniques of pressing and manipulation. Your partner lies in the supine position (on the back), and each leg is held straight and thoroughly pressed using the palms and thumbs. Ensure that all the the Sen/Meridians are equally stimulated along the entire length of the leg.

In the second part of Lesson Two, the leg is placed in every position possible to give complete access to the Sen/Meridians (see right). The techniques are applied first to one leg and then repeated on the other.

SEN/MERIDIANS ON THE LEGS

Energy balance in the leg Sen/Meridians is essential for energy balance in the spine. Throughout the bodywork, Thais place much emphasis on the legs as energy flow through them strongly affects the health of the whole body. There's no definitive agreement as to the exact course of the Sen lines, but the Thais consider there to be three lines on the inside and three on the outside of each leg, corresponding with the Chinese Meridians.

INNER SEN/YIN MERIDIANS

Sen/Meridians on the inside of the leg are located as follows:

Sen 1 Chinese Spleen Meridian Starts on the medial big toe, passes under the inner ankle bone and along the inner edge of the shin bone to just beneath the knee (SP 9) and then up the inner thigh to the top of the groin.

Sen 2 Chinese Liver Meridian Starts on the lateral big toe and runs in front of the inner ankle bone, then behind and roughly parallel with Sen 1/Spleen Meridian up the calf and through the medial side of the knee to the groin.

Sen 3 Chinese Kidney Meridian Starts under the sole of the foot (K 1) and runs between the Achilles tendon and the inner ankle bone (K 3), roughly parallel and behind Sen 2/Liver Meridian up the calf to the back of the knee and to the groin.

— Sen 1

— Sen 2

— Sen 3

OUTER SEN/YANG MERIDIANS

Sen/Meridians on the outside of the leg are located as follows:

Sen 1 Chinese Stomach Meridian Runs from the lateral side of the second toe, through the centre of the ankle (ST 41) to the lateral knee eye parallel to the crest of the tibia, up the thigh, in line with the outer edge of the patella, and to the front of the hip (ST 31).

Sen 2 Chinese Gall Bladder Meridian Runs from the lateral fourth toe, through the outer ankle (GB 40), up the side of the leg one thumb-width behind Sen 1/Stomach Meridian, and runs roughly parallel with it towards the hip joint.

Sen 3 Chinese Bladder Meridian Runs from the side of the fifth toe, between the Achilles tendon and the outer ankle bone, and up the leg on the midline to the buttocks (BL 36).

This illustration shows the three inner Sen/Yin Meridians and the three outer Sen/Yang Meridians. Part of the third one is under the straight leg and cannot be seen in this position.

NOTE: Chinese Leg Yin Meridians start on the feet and end on the chest. Chinese Leg Yang Meridians start on the head and end on the toes.

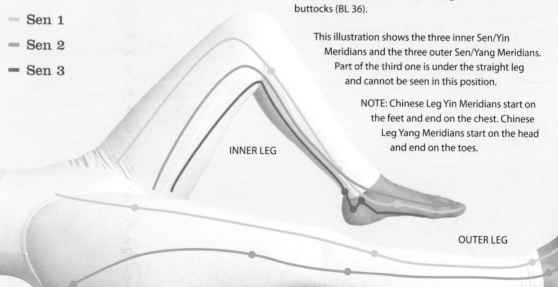

INNER LEG

OUTER LEG

NOTE: The Liver Meridian has been slightly altered to match the Sen 2 and run behind the Spleen Meridian.

PRESSING THE LEGS

1 PRESSING THE INNER FEET & LEGS

Palm press both feet and ankles, rocking them both outwards or
each alternately from side to side. Continue pressing up the inner
legs to the groin and back again. Don't press the knees, but, using
a light circular motion, rub them with cupped hands. Repeat several
times. Always maintain an even rhythm to promote relaxation.

2 PRESSING THE INNER RIGHT LEG

Touch method one: palm pressing
Kneel between your partner's legs, facing the inside of the right
leg. Starting above and below the right knee, palm press with
both hands simultaneously up the thigh and down the calf. You
could also start just above the ankle, using both hands side by
side, and gradually palm press up the leg and down again. Repeat,
palm pressing each Sen/Meridian.

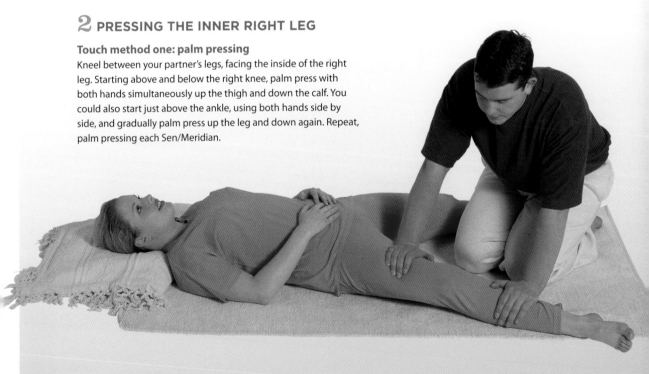

3 PRESSING THE OUTER RIGHT LEG

Change position to outside the right leg and repeat the palming and thumbing sequences on the outer Sen lines/ST and GB Meridians. Press-knead ST 36, ST 31, GB 34 and GB 31. Repeat steps 2 and 3 on the left leg.

HEALING BENEFITS

Improves energy flow in the ST and GB Meridians and relieves sciatic pain.

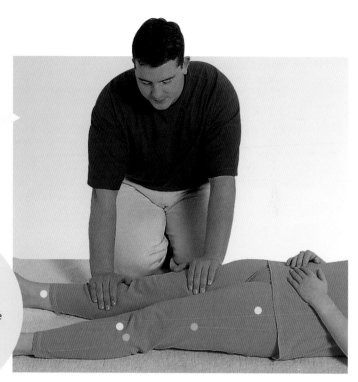

HEALING BENEFITS

Releases myofascia and stimulates energy flow in the Sen/SP, K and LIV Meridians.

Touch method two: thumb pressing
Using the thumb walking technique, thumb up Sen line 1 (SP Meridian) to your partner's knee, down line 2 (K Meridian) to the ankle, up line 3 (LIV Meridian) to the knee and down line 2 again. Repeat this sequence several times. Press-knead K 3, SP 6 and SP 9. When you've finished thumbing the lower leg, move up and repeat the sequence on the upper energy pathways, spanning the knee to the groin. Finish by palming your partner's leg once more.

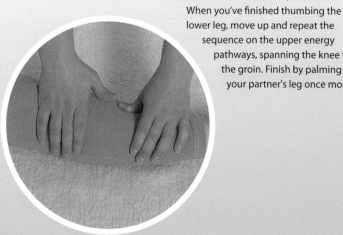

MUSCLES STRETCHED & PRESSED

1 **Pressing the inner feet & legs**
   Stretched: SOLEUS, GASTROCNEMIUS, ADDUCTORS

2 **Pressing the inner right leg**
   Stretched: SOLEUS, GASTROCNEMIUS, ADDUCTORS

3 **Pressing the outer right leg**
   Stretched: PERONEUS LONGUS, GASTROCNEMIUS, BICEPS FEMORIS, VASTUS LATERALIS

MASSAGING THE RIGHT LEG ONLY

1 PRESSING THE LEG IN THE TREE POSITION

Touch method one

Place your partner's right leg in the tree position, keeping the foot tucked against the straight left leg. Support the left hip with your right hand while you palm up and down the inner Sen channels of the bent leg with a slight rocking action. Don't hurry your movements – the presses should be sustained.

HEALING BENEFITS

Aids flexibility and relaxation of the knee and hip.

Stimulates the energy pathways that affect the urinogenital organs.

Touch method two: thumb pressing

Proceed from palming to thumbing, which is carried out in exactly the same way as described earlier (see page 45).

HEALING BENEFITS

Even the stiffest hips and knees can be coaxed into a state of relaxation and release.

Especially helpful for those who experience spasms and stiffness in the adductor muscles of the thigh.

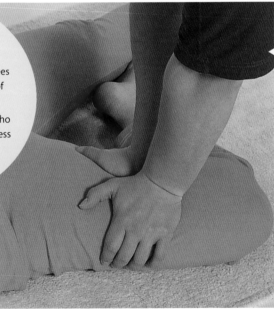

2 BUTTERFLY PRESSING THE LEG IN THE TREE POSITION

Slightly alter your position, facing directly towards your partner's flexed knee. Using both hands simultaneously, butterfly press the entire length of the flexed leg.

MUSCLES STRETCHED & PRESSED

1 Pressing the leg in the tree position

2 Butterfly pressing the leg in the tree position

3 Foot pressing the leg in the tree position

Stretched: ADDUCTORS, SARTORIUS
Pressed: ADDUCTORS, SOLEUS, GRACILIS,
SEMIMEMBRANOSUS, SEMITENDINOSUS,
GASTROCNEMIUS

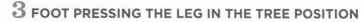

HEALING BENEFITS

Tight and spasming thigh adductor muscles respond well to the foot pressing methods.

3 FOOT PRESSING THE LEG IN THE TREE POSITION

Touch method one

Assume a kneeling stance, balancing yourself by lightly leaning on your partner's thigh and knee. Use your right foot to massage the bent leg. Press carefully and deeply all along the thigh with your toes and the ball of your foot. Rock forwards slowly to find the necessary pressure.

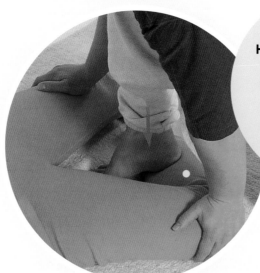

HEALING BENEFITS

Helps tight or spasming calf muscles to relax, stimulating blood and lymph flow.

Treats calf muscle injured through sport.

Touch method two

With a slight change in your position, heel press along your partner's calf muscles using your body weight to achieve controlled pressure. Heel press SP 6 and SP 9.

HEALING BENEFITS
STEPS 4, 5, 6 & 7

These powerful techniques relax the inner hamstrings, enhance knee mobility and boost Sen/SP, K and LIV energies.

Some types of sciatica are eased.

Useful for treating hamstrings injured through sport.

4 SINGLE GRAPE PRESS

Place the sole of your left foot against your partner's right thigh just behind and above the knee. Hold both feet and lean back while you press up the thigh towards the groin and back again, as if you were treading grapes.

5 SINGLE GRAPE PRESS & TWISTED VINE

Now tuck your left foot snugly behind your partner's knee and cross the right leg across your shin, tucking the toes behind your knee to give the impression of a twisted vine. Hold your partner's heel to keep the foot in this position while you bring your right foot across and place it under the right thigh. Now press progressively with your right foot towards the groin and back again, keeping a steady, slow rhythm and firm pressure. Repeat several times.

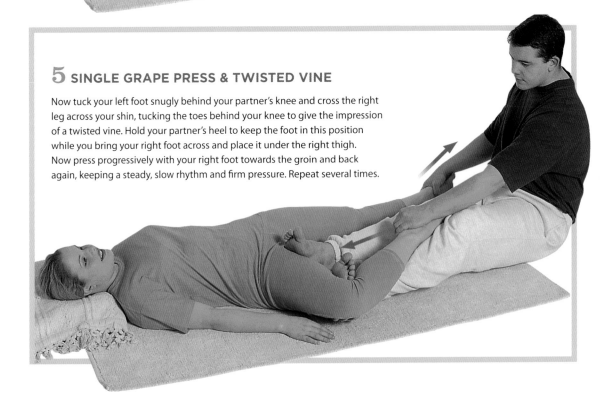

MUSCLES STRETCHED & PRESSED

4 Single grape press
Stretched: ADDUCTORS, SARTORIUS, GRACILIS
Pressed: ADDUCTORS, HAMSTRINGS

5 Single grape press & twisted vine
Stretched: ADDUCTORS, SARTORIUS, GRACILIS
Pressed: ADDUCTORS, HAMSTRINGS

6 Double grape press
Stretched: ADDUCTORS, SARTORIUS, GRACILIS
Pressed: ADDUCTORS, HAMSTRINGS

7 Grape press & squeeze
Stretched: THIGH ADDUCTORS, SARTORIUS, GRACILIS
Pressed: ADDUCTORS, HAMSTRINGS

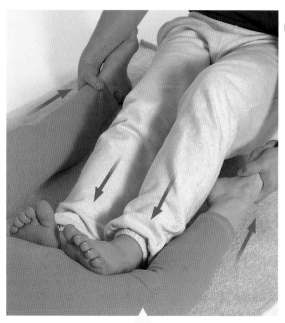

6 DOUBLE GRAPE PRESS

Release your partner's right foot from the locked position but continue to hold both ankles. Now press up and down the right thigh, using your feet alternately. Repeat several times.

7 GRAPE PRESS & SQUEEZE

Now place your right foot on your partner's inner thigh and slide your left foot under the leg. Squeeze and press both the inner and outer thighs together. Start at the knee, pressing and squeezing up the thigh and then back to the knee. Lean your body back with each press and squeeze.

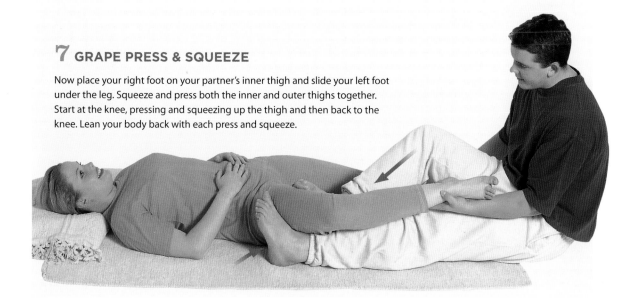

HEALING BENEFITS

Promotes limb relaxation and increased hip and knee flexibility.

Stimulates the energy pathways.

8 Z-STOP

Keep your feet tucked in snugly behind your partner's knee and cross the lower leg across both your shins. The leg will become bent at a sharply acute angle that resembles a Z-shape (left). Slide forwards a little to grasp the front surface of your partner's thigh and pull it towards you. Pull alternately with both hands along the length of the thigh (below).

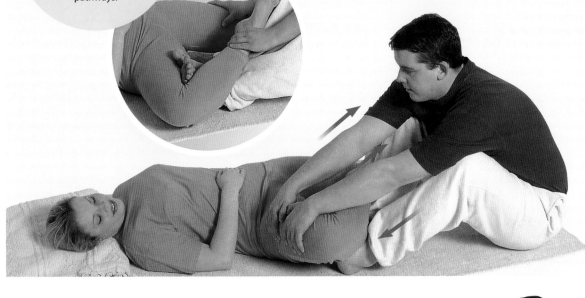

9 PULLING THE CALF

Touch method one

Lift your partner's flexed leg and lock the foot between your knees. Place your hands behind the calf so that your fingertips are pressing into the Bladder Meridian at BL 57 and pull towards you, rocking gently backwards. Repeat at different positions along the calf.

Touch method two

Place your left hand behind the upper calf muscles. Squeeze and drag them to your left. Change hands and repeat in the opposite direction.

HEALING BENEFITS

Stimulates energy flow in Sen/Bladder Meridian to loosen fibrotic connective tissue.

Good for football and rugby players.

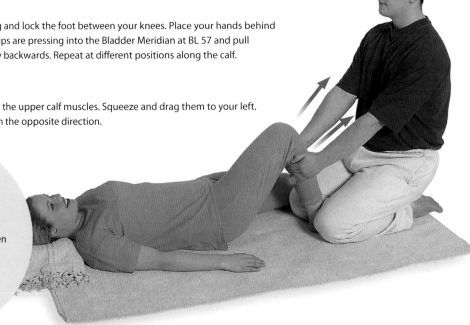

10 PRESSING THE UPPER THIGH

Touch method one
Interlock the fingers of your hands across your partner's thigh, just above the knee. Squeeze firmly with the heels of your hands to cover the full length of the upper leg to the groin. Repeat several times.

Touch method two
Pummel inner and outer thighs and calves at the same time. Repeat several times.

MUSCLES STRETCHED & PRESSED

8 Z-stop
Stretched: QUADRICEPS, ADDUCTORS
Pressed: HAMSTRINGS, ADDUCTORS, QUADRICEPS

9 Pulling the calf
Pressed: GASTROCNEMIUS, SOLEUS

10 Pressing the upper thigh
Pressed: QUADRICEPS, SARTORIUS, GRACILIS, SEMIMEMBRANOSUS

11 Chest to foot thigh pressing
Stretched: GLUTEUS MAXIMUS, QUADRICEPS, ERECTOR SPINA
Pressed: HAMSTRINGS

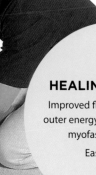

HEALING BENEFITS
Improved flow in the inner and outer energy pathways to release myofascial adhesions.
Eases sciatica.

11 CHEST TO FOOT THIGH PRESSING

Lift your partner's right leg and place the foot on your chest. Support the knee with your right hand and, with your left hand, press firmly into the thigh muscles. Press BL 37 and BL 36. Gently rock your partner in a forwards-and-backwards motion as you press up and down the thigh muscle.

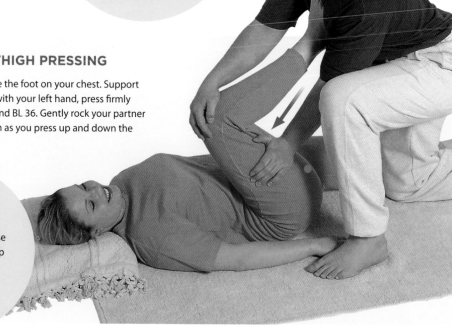

HEALING BENEFITS
Gives myofascial release to the hamstring group of muscles.
Eases hip pain and sciatica.

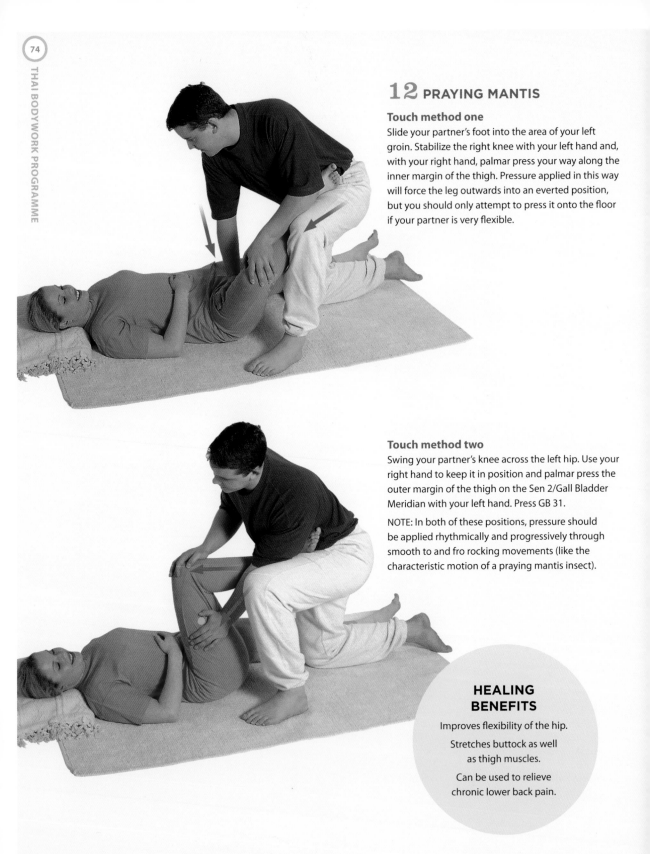

12 PRAYING MANTIS

Touch method one

Slide your partner's foot into the area of your left groin. Stabilize the right knee with your left hand and, with your right hand, palmar press your way along the inner margin of the thigh. Pressure applied in this way will force the leg outwards into an everted position, but you should only attempt to press it onto the floor if your partner is very flexible.

Touch method two

Swing your partner's knee across the left hip. Use your right hand to keep it in position and palmar press the outer margin of the thigh on the Sen 2/Gall Bladder Meridian with your left hand. Press GB 31.

NOTE: In both of these positions, pressure should be applied rhythmically and progressively through smooth to and fro rocking movements (like the characteristic motion of a praying mantis insect).

HEALING BENEFITS

Improves flexibility of the hip.

Stretches buttock as well as thigh muscles.

Can be used to relieve chronic lower back pain.

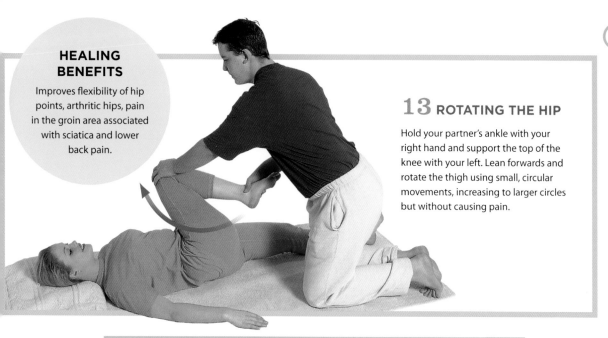

HEALING BENEFITS

Improves flexibility of hip points, arthritic hips, pain in the groin area associated with sciatica and lower back pain.

13 ROTATING THE HIP

Hold your partner's ankle with your right hand and support the top of the knee with your left. Lean forwards and rotate the thigh using small, circular movements, increasing to larger circles but without causing pain.

MUSCLES STRETCHED & PRESSED

12 Praying mantis
Stretched: ADDUCTORS, GLUTEALS, ERECTOR SPINAE, QUADRICEPS PIRIFORMIS
Pressed: SEMIMEMBRANOSUS, SEMITENDINOSUS, BICEPS FEMORIS, VASTUS LATERALIS

13 Rotating the hip
Stretched: GLUTEUS MAXIMUS, PIRIFORMIS, SACROSPINALIS, QUADRICEPSS

14 Kneeing the thigh
Pressed: HAMSTRINGS

HEALING BENEFITS

Good for the treatment of tense and spasming hamstrings caused by sports injury, repetitive strain, back pain and sciatica.

14 KNEEING THE THIGH

Lift your partner's right leg and place your left knee against the back of the thigh at BL 37. Hold the heel and knee and firmly pull the thigh against your knee. Relax the pulling force, lower your knee slightly and pull again. Repeat several times to knee-press the full length of the thigh on the Bladder Meridian, pressing BL 36 and BL 37.

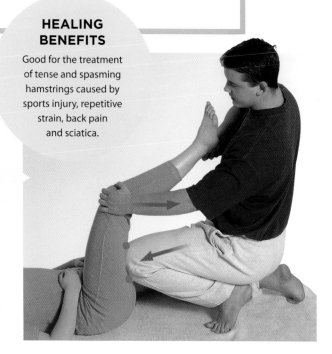

MUSCLES STRETCHED & PRESSED

15 Pressing thigh to calf
Stretched: ANTERIOR TIBIALIS
Pressed: GASTROCNEMIUS, SOLEUS,
POSTERIOR TIBIALIS

16 Arm cracker
Stretched: ANTERIOR TIBIALIS,
ANKLE AND FOOT FLEXORS
Pressed: HAMSTRINGS,
GASTROCNEMIUS

17 Flexing & stretching the leg
Stretched: GASTROCNEMIUS,
SOLEUS (leg extended); HAMSTRINGS,
GLUTEUS (leg flexed)

18 Pressing foot to thigh
Pressed: HAMSTRINGS

15 PRESSING THIGH TO CALF

Place the calf of your partner's right leg across your left thigh. Press down on the knee and foot to firmly press BL 57 on the Bladder Meridian. Adjust the position of your partner's leg to press up and down the whole calf.

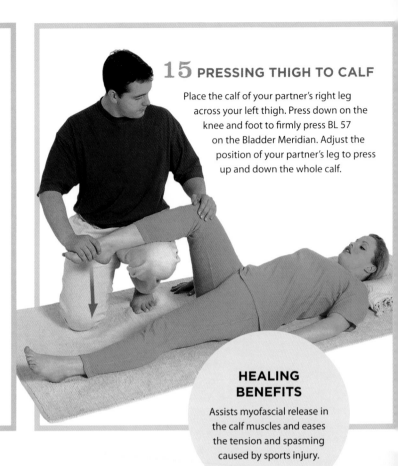

HEALING BENEFITS

Assists myofascial release in the calf muscles and eases the tension and spasming caused by sports injury.

16 ARM CRACKER

Tuck your left wrist and forearm tightly in behind your partner's knee. Now press the foot downwards to give a very strong stretch across the trapped arm. Repeat two to three times.

HEALING BENEFITS

Treats knee pain, spasming hamstring and calf muscles.

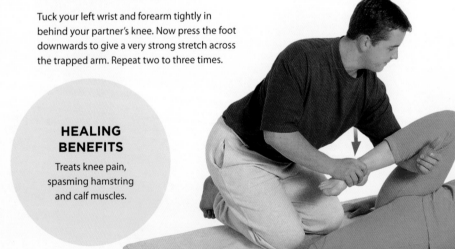

HEALING BENEFITS

Opens the hip, knee and ankle joints.

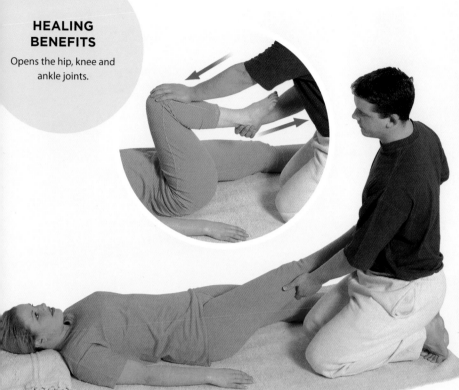

17 FLEXING & STRETCHING THE LEG

Grasp your partner's right heel underneath and support the side of the knee. Flex the leg at the knee by pushing the knee and then sharply extend it to maximum effect by pulling the heel, assisted by a quick pull on the knee. Repeat the exercise several times.

CAUTION

This technique must not be practised on those who have had any kind of knee or hip surgery.

18 PRESSING FOOT TO THIGH

Grasp your partner's right foot. Place your right foot diagonally with the arch across the back of the thigh on the Bladder Meridian. Lean back, pulling the leg towards you to generate a strong, sustained pressure on the hamstrings. Release the pressure, move the foot to a lower position and pull. Repeat several times to cover the whole of the thigh.

HEALING BENEFITS

Treats sports injuries to the hamstrings, lower back, hip pain and some forms of sciatica.

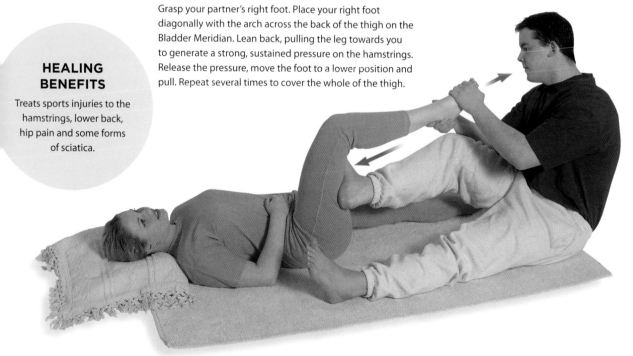

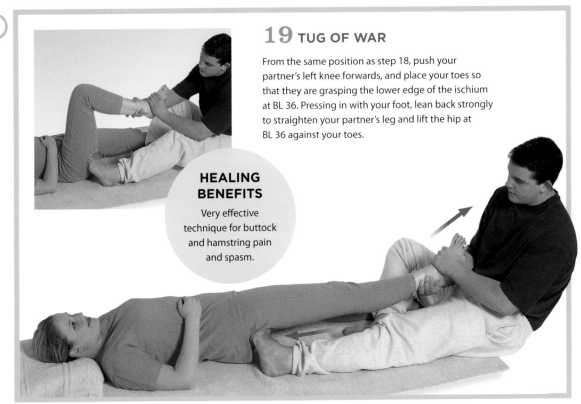

19 TUG OF WAR

From the same position as step 18, push your partner's left knee forwards, and place your toes so that they are grasping the lower edge of the ischium at BL 36. Pressing in with your foot, lean back strongly to straighten your partner's leg and lift the hip at BL 36 against your toes.

HEALING BENEFITS

Very effective technique for buttock and hamstring pain and spasm.

HEALING BENEFITS

Stretches the quadriceps, hips, knees and ankles.

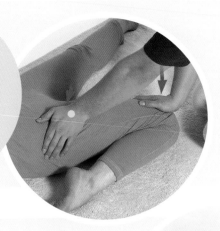

20 PRESSING THE TURNED-IN LEG

If your partner is flexible enough, position the right leg with the thigh turned in and the lower leg everted. If not, use your own knee to support your partner's knee. Single or butterfly press the outer margin of the thigh. Press ST 31.

21 PRESSING THE LEANING LEG

Reposition your partner's right leg so that it now leans against the straight one. Palmar press the exposed thigh area several times. Finish by placing one hand over the hip joint and the other on the knee, and press very firmly. Hold for at least ten seconds.

HEALING BENEFITS

Loosens the hip joint. Stimulates energy flow in the outer Sen/Gall Bladder Meridian to relieve lower back and leg pain. Knead GB 31 and GB 34.

22 ROCKING THE HIP

Place your partner's right leg over the left and locate the foot in position by placing the arch of your right foot lightly across the toes. Tuck your left hand under the right upper hip while pushing the right knee gently towards the mat on your partner's left side. Establish a to-and-fro rocking movement, aiming to get the knee closer to the floor with each rock.

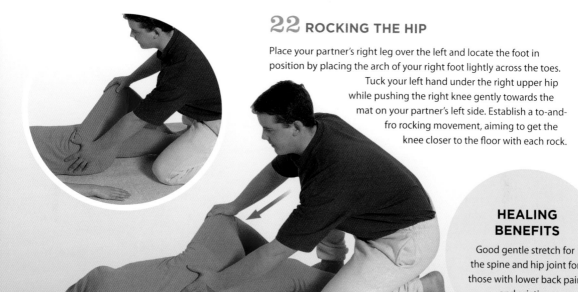

HEALING BENEFITS

Good gentle stretch for the spine and hip joint for those with lower back pain and sciatica.

CAUTION

When pressing your partner's shoulder down, this must be done carefully with full awareness of your partner's reactions.

23 SHOULDER TO OPPOSITE KNEE SPINAL TWIST

As you finish the previous technique, hold your partner's right knee down in its most extreme position, place your left hand on the front of the right shoulder and press smoothly and firmly. Hold for at least ten seconds.

HEALING BENEFITS

Treats lumbar and hip pain.

Increases spinal mobility.

MUSCLES STRETCHED & PRESSED

19 **Tug of war**
   Stretched: ANTERIOR TIBIALIS, QUADRICEPS
   Pressed: HAMSTRINGS, GRACILIS

20 **Pressing the turned-in leg**
   Stretched: QUADRICEPS, SARTORIUS
   Pressed: VASTUS LATERALIS, VASTUS INTERMEDIUS, RECTUS FEMORIS

21 **Pressing the leaning leg**
   Pressed: VASTUS LATERALIS, BICEPS FEMORIS, TENSOR FASCIAE LATAE

22 **Rocking the hip**
   Stretched: QUADRATUS LUMBORUM, PIRIFORMIS
   Pressed: VASTUS LATERALIS, BICEPS FEMORIS, TENSOR FASCIAE LATAE

23 **Shoulder to opposite knee spinal twist**
   Stretched: QUADRATUS LUMBORUM, PIRIFORMIS
   Pressed: VASTUS LATERALIS, RECTUS FEMORIS, BICEPS FEMORIS

24 STRETCHING THE CROSSED LEG HORIZONTALLY

Move to the other side of your partner and extend the right leg across the left hip, holding the right ankle and pressing down on the right hip. Press GB 29, GB 30 and BL 54. Stretch the leg by pushing it towards the head with your knee. Keep the leg straight and only stretch as far as is comfortable.

HEALING BENEFITS

Improves hip flexibility and eases tension in the buttocks and hamstrings.

Treats lower back pain and sciatica.

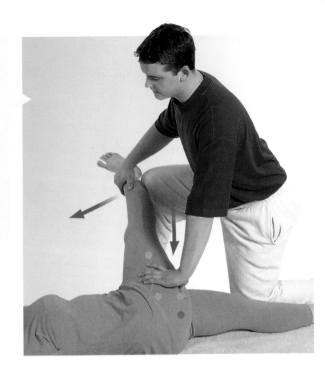

25 PRESSING IN THE SPLITS POSITION

Spread your partner's legs apart as far as is comfortable and hold them in this position with your feet. Palmar and thumb press the inner Sen lines/Spleen, Kidney and Liver Meridians in the lower leg and the thigh. Knead SP 6 and SP 9.

HEALING BENEFITS

Eases groin pain and treats injuries to the thigh adductors.

Helps lymphatic drainage from the lower leg.

MUSCLES STRETCHED & PRESSED

24 Stretching the crossed leg horizontally
Stretched: GASTROCNEMIUS, BICEPS FEMORIS, PIRIFORMIS, GLUTEUS MAXIMUS, SOLEUS
Pressed: GLUTEUS MAXIMUS

25 Pressing in the splits position
Stretched: ADDUCTORS, GRACILIS, GASTROCNEMIUS, HAMSTRINGS
Pressed: ALL THE STRETCHED MUSCLES

26 Swinging the leg in the splits position
Stretched: ADDUCTORS, GRACILIS, GASTROCNEMIUS, HAMSTRINGS
Pressed: all the stretched muscles

27 Half lotus press
Stretched: ADDUCTORS, GRACILIS
Pressed: ADDUCTORS, GRACILIS

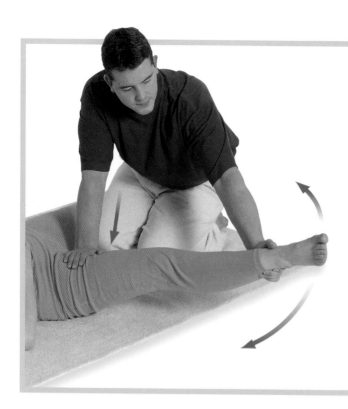

HEALING BENEFITS

Treats pain in the thigh adductors and groin.

Aids hip mobility.

26 SWINGING THE LEG IN THE SPLITS POSITION

Support the top of your partner's thigh with your right hand and grasp the heel with your left hand. Swing the leg out to the side as far as is comfortable. Then swing the leg backwards and forwards several times.

27 HALF LOTUS PRESS

Touch method one
Lift your partner's leg into a half lotus position, with the right ankle lying above the left knee. If your partner is very stiff, you'll need to support the flexed leg across your knee. With your right hand holding down the left thigh, press up and down the inner energy Sen/Meridians of the flexed leg with a rocking motion.

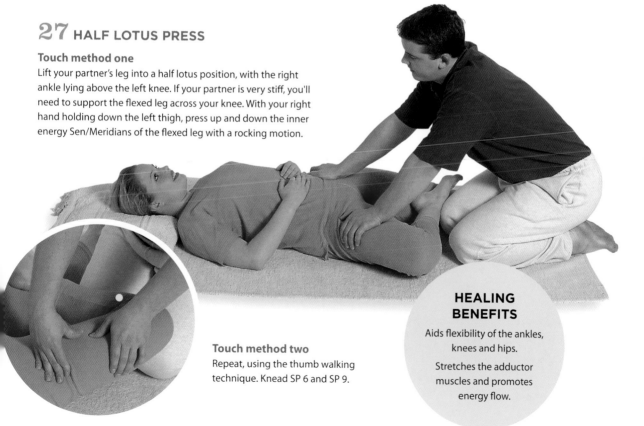

Touch method two
Repeat, using the thumb walking technique. Knead SP 6 and SP 9.

HEALING BENEFITS

Aids flexibility of the ankles, knees and hips.

Stretches the adductor muscles and promotes energy flow.

28 HALF LOTUS HIP ROCK

With your partner still in the half lotus position, lift the straightened left leg across your right thigh. Holding the foot and knee of the flexed right leg, rock the knee to and fro sideways.

HEALING BENEFITS

Improves knee and hip mobility and treats lower lumbar, sacral and sciatic pain.

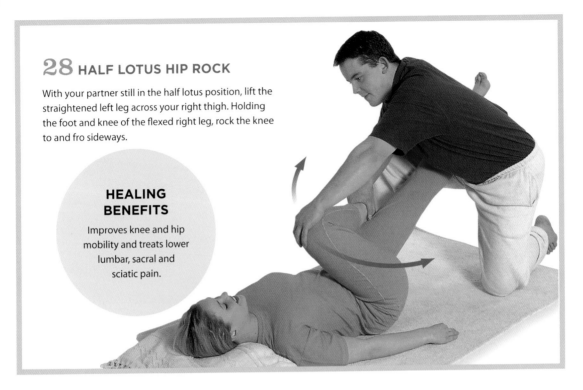

29 HALF LOTUS BACK ROCK & ROLL

Still in the half lotus, hold your partner's right heel and push the right leg forwards over the head while stabilizing her buttocks with your other hand. Establish a to and fro rocking action.

HEALING BENEFITS

Eases back pain and improves back and hip mobility.

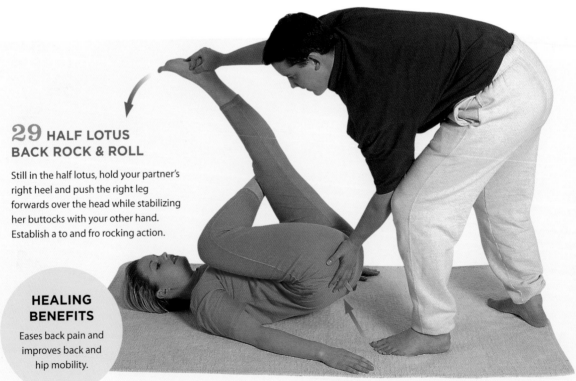

HEALING BENEFITS

Treats lower back pain and sciatica and improves mobility in the hip and knee.

30 VERTICAL HALF LOTUS THIGH PRESS

Maintaining the half lotus, lift your partner's straightened left leg into a vertical position, supporting the ankle against your shoulder. Hold the ankle of the right foot and palmar press the exposed thigh from BL 36 to the knee, keeping your arm straight and rocking forwards with each press.

31 CORKSCREW

With your partner's right leg still firmly in the half lotus, hold the left leg vertically. Move forwards and step over the flexed right leg with your left leg. Place your left foot so that your toes are under your partner's armpit and keep your knees slightly flexed. Tuck your right leg against the outer margin of the vertical leg and use it to support that leg. By gradually straightening your left leg you will exert a backwards pressure on the flexed leg and this will generate a twisting action on the hips and lower back. Knead the sole and the heel of the left foot with your right elbow. Elbow knead K 1.

MUSCLES STRETCHED & PRESSED

28 Half lotus hip rock
Stretched: HAMSTRINGS (straight leg); GLUTEUS MAXIMUS (flexed leg)

29 Half lotus back rock & roll
Stretched: HAMSTRINGS (straight leg); ADDUCTORS, GRACILIS (flexed leg)

30 Vertical half lotus thigh press
Stretched: GLUTEUS MAXIMUS (bent leg); SOLEUS, GASTROCNEMIUS, HAMSTRINGS (straight leg)

31 Corkscrew
Stretched: ADDUCTORS, VASTUS MEDIALIS, GRACILIS (flexed leg); GASTROCNEMIUS, SOLEUS, HAMSTRINGS (straight leg)

CAUTION

Be careful not to overdo the twisting action. If your partner is very stiff, stand further back with your right leg and only raise and push the straight leg as far as it will comfortably go without twisting the hips with your other leg. Don't use on elderly people.

HEALING BENEFITS

Increases hip and lower back flexibility.

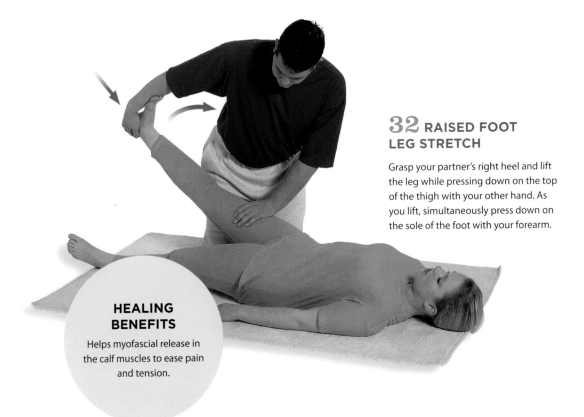

32 RAISED FOOT LEG STRETCH

Grasp your partner's right heel and lift the leg while pressing down on the top of the thigh with your other hand. As you lift, simultaneously press down on the sole of the foot with your forearm.

HEALING BENEFITS

Helps myofascial release in the calf muscles to ease pain and tension.

33 VERTICAL LEG STRETCH

Raise your partner's right leg to as near vertical as is comfortable and support the foot against the front of your shoulder. Keep the leg straight, with your right hand across the knee. Place your knee lightly across the left thigh on ST 31 to hold it down. Gently push the leg forwards several times, each time slightly increasing the stretch.

HEALING BENEFITS

Relaxes tense or spasming calf and hamstring muscles resulting from sports injuries, sciatica and back pain.

CAUTION

Take care when kneeling along the top of your partner's thigh.

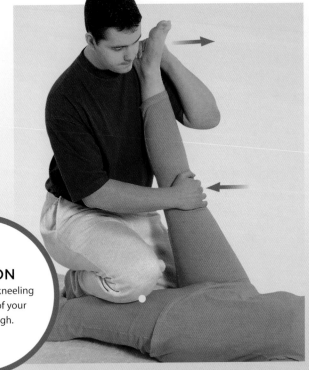

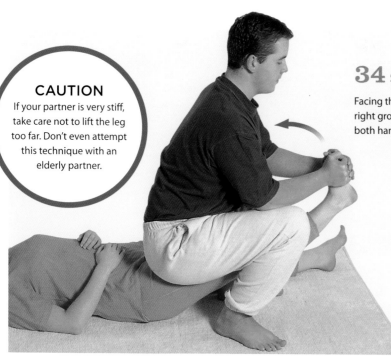

CAUTION
If your partner is very stiff, take care not to lift the leg too far. Don't even attempt this technique with an elderly partner.

34 SEESAW LEG STRETCH

Facing the feet, sit very lightly on your partner's right groin on ST 31. Grasp the right foot with both hands and lift the leg towards you.

HEALING BENEFITS

Treats spasming calf and hamstring muscles. ST 31 energizes the front hip.

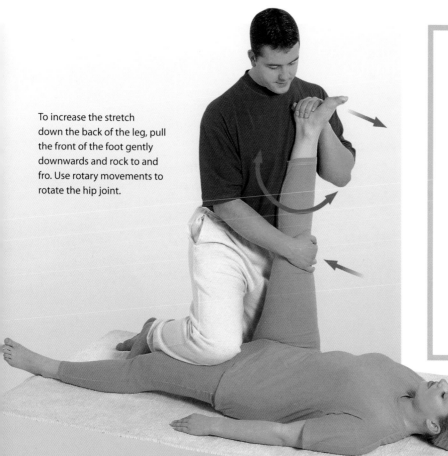

To increase the stretch down the back of the leg, pull the front of the foot gently downwards and rock to and fro. Use rotary movements to rotate the hip joint.

MUSCLES STRETCHED & PRESSED

32 Raised foot leg stretch
Stretched: HAMSTRINGS, PERONEUS LONGUS, GASTROCNEMIUS, SOLEUS

33 Vertical leg stretch
Stretched: HAMSTRINGS, GASTROCNEMIUS, SOLEUS, PERONEUS LONGUS (foot pressed down)

34 Seesaw leg stretch
Stretched: GASTROCNEMIUS, HAMSTRINGS
Pressed: QUADRICEPS

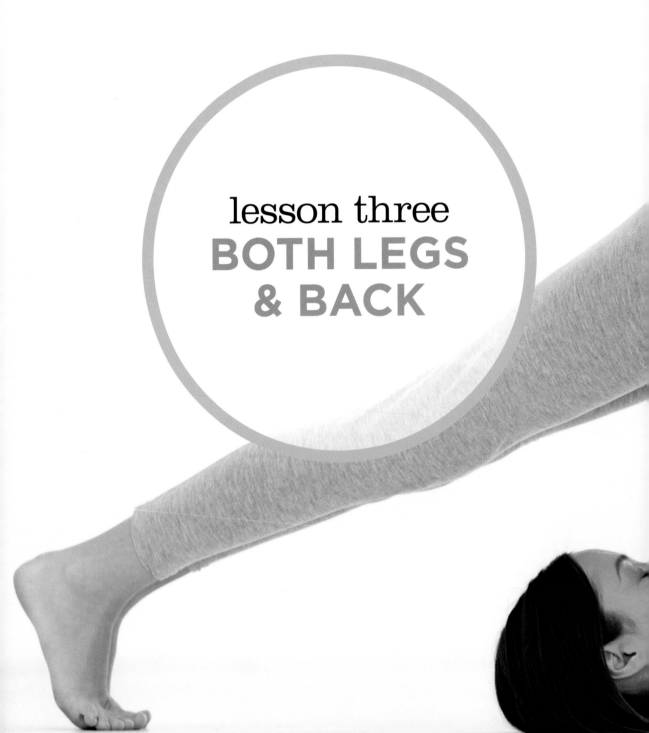

lesson three
BOTH LEGS & BACK

The aim of this lesson is to stimulate energy flow between the trunk and legs. A healthy backbone needs to bend and rotate in many directions. Pain in the lumbar area is common and can be caused not only by sports injuries but also by poor posture. Acute pain can be triggered by sudden twisting of the waist or lifting heavy loads. Many of the techniques featured here provide powerful muscle stretches that can correct postural imbalances and relax spasming muscles, thereby relieving back pain.

MUSCLES STRETCHED & PRESSED

1 Pressing the inner feet & legs
   Stretched: ADDUCTORS

2 Leg blood stop
   Stretched: ADDUCTORS

3 Bow & arrow spinal twist
   Stretched: QUADRATUS LUMBORUM,
   RHOMBOIDEUS MAJOR & MINOR,
   LEVATOR SCAPULAE, TRAPEZIUS,
   ERECTOR SPINAE, ILIACUS, PSOAS MAJOR

4 Rotating the hips
   Stretched: GLUTEUS MAXIMUS,
   QUADRICEPS (slight stretch),
   QUADRATUS LUMBORUM

1 PRESSING THE INNER FEET & LEGS

Repeat the first technique in Lesson Two (see page 64). Re-establishing contact with the feet encourages a sense of body and mind integration and general well-being. As the inner Sen start on the feet and legs, pressing the inner legs stimulates energy flow between the legs and trunk.

HEALING BENEFITS

When blood flow into the legs is interrupted, the entire circulation, including lymphatic drainage, is reduced or completely stopped. The swift rush of blood into the legs is accompanied by a sudden spread of warmth down to the feet as full circulation is restored. After this treatment, the legs feel very light.

2 LEG BLOOD STOP

Your partner should be lying supine in a totally relaxed position with the legs slightly apart. Kneel and palm up both thighs until your palms reach the groin. Press down on the three leg Sen/Inner Meridians and adjust your hands until you feel the blood pulsing through the femoral arteries beneath the heels of your palms.

   Now lift your body by straightening your legs or arching your buttocks. This will focus your weight on your palms, thus increasing pressure on your partner's arteries to restrict the flow of blood through them. Hold for thirty to fifty seconds

CAUTION

Don't attempt this technique on those with any kind of circulatory problem such as varicose veins, high blood pressure or heart disease.

3 BOW & ARROW SPINAL TWIST

Tuck your right heel behind your partner's left flexed knee and grasp and pull the left forearm towards you (below), keeping the left leg firmly located on the mat. Now lean across and grasp under the left shoulder (inset right) with both hands and pull carefully towards you. Pull the shoulder and along your partner's side with alternate hand movements, which should be kept slow and rhythmical.

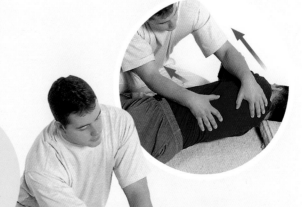

HEALING BENEFITS

Treats lower back pain, improves spinal mobility and aligns the spine.

CAUTION

Don't use on those who have had surgery on the lower back.

4 ROTATING THE HIPS

Lift your partner's flexed legs so that the knees are directly over the abdomen. Your legs should be astride the ankles, with your hands just below the knees. Starting with just a small amplitude rotation of the knees, gradually increase. Keep both knees together. Rotate about fifteen times in each direction.

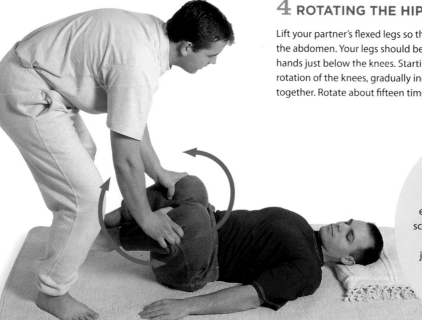

HEALING BENEFITS

Has a soothing effect on those who experience stiffness in the hip region, sciatica and lower back pain. In addition to the rotation imposed on the hip joint, a twisting action on the lumbar vertebrae also occurs, which relaxes muscles in the hip.

HEALING BENEFITS
STEPS 5 & 6

Essential for those suffering from lower back pain and sciatica. These techniques can also be used on those who suffer from varicose veins.

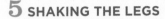

5 SHAKING THE LEGS

Grasp your partner's ankles, lean back slightly to create traction and shake the legs up and down rapidly with a small-amplitude movement. Shake the legs ten to twenty times.

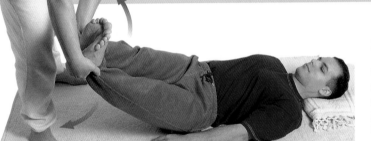

6 SWINGING THE LEGS

Now hold your partner's legs at the ankles and swing from side to side at least fifteen times. Start with small, slow swings that gradually get bigger and faster.

7 ROCKING & ROLLING THE BACK

Use your right hand to hold your partner's heels so that both legs are straight. Push the feet forwards over the head, using your other hand to help lift the buttocks. Determine how far your partner can comfortably roll back, and then rock and roll to and fro up to this limit. The movement requires a very smooth and controlled rocking action from you.

CAUTION
Take care not to overstretch anyone you're giving massage to for the first time.

HEALING BENEFITS

Helps to ease middle and upper back pain.

8 THE PLOUGH

Spread your partner's legs out into an open V-shape and step through them to adopt a new position astride the body with your feet tucked under the armpits. Bend your knees slightly towards the midline, increase the V angle between the legs and draw them around your knees. Press the feet together and then press lightly downwards. Hold for a few seconds, then open the legs again, draw them back around your legs and push the feet forwards and down a little further in the direction of your partner's head. In a very flexible person the feet will touch the floor. Repeat this until you find the most extreme position that's comfortable. Hold the position for at least ten seconds.

HEALING BENEFITS

Aids mobility of the hip joints, lower back and sacrum.

A gentle to and fro rocking motion (as shown in first image, top left) relieves lower back pain and can be done on the elderly.

MUSCLES STRETCHED & PRESSED

7 Rocking & rolling the back
Stretched: ERECTOR SPINAE, GASTROCNEMIUS

8 The plough
Stretched: ADDUCTORS, SOLEUS, HAMSTRINGS, GLUTEUS MAXIMUS, ERECTOR SPINAE

9 KNEEING THE BACKS OF THE THIGHS

As your partner is released from the previous position, retain your hold on the feet and step back through the legs again. Hold the feet so that the legs are slightly bent. Using your body weight, press both knees into the backs of your partner's thighs on BL 36 while pushing the feet forwards. Press progressively along the thigh.

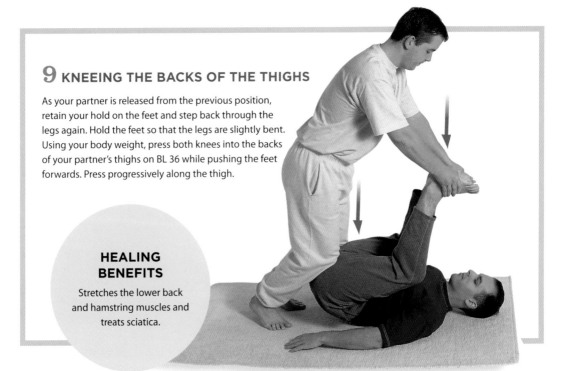

HEALING BENEFITS

Stretches the lower back and hamstring muscles and treats sciatica.

10 KNEEING THE BUTTOCKS

Lift your partner's buttocks off the mat and support with both hands while you knead around BL 54 deeply with circular movements of your knees.

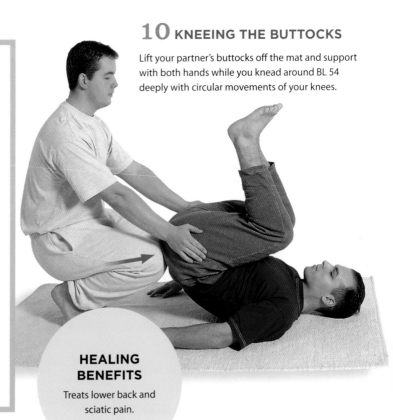

MUSCLES STRETCHED & PRESSED

9 Kneeing the backs of the thighs
Stretched: ERECTOR SPINAE, GLUTEUS MAXIMUS
Pressed: HAMSTRINGS, GLUTEUS MAXIMUS (lower part)

10 Kneeing the buttocks
Stretched: ERECTOR SPINAE, GLUTEUS MAXIMUS
Pressed: GLUTEUS MAXIMUS

11 Shinning the thighs
Stretched: GLUTEUS MAXIMUS
Pressed: HAMSTRINGS

12 The half bridge
Stretched: QUADRICEPS, RECTUS ABDOMINIS, ERECTOR SPINAE

HEALING BENEFITS

Treats lower back and sciatic pain.

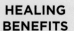

HEALING BENEFITS

Another excellent treatment for sciatica; also very effective for myofascial release around the hamstrings, particularly for those who do a lot of sport.

11 SHINNING THE THIGHS

Good balance is required for the correct execution of this technique. Bend your partner's right leg into a right angle so that the thigh is lying against the abdomen. Hold the other leg outwards and then lean your left knee inwards so that your shin presses against the thigh. Shin progressively along the entire length of your partner's thigh on the Gall Bladder Meridian with a to and fro rocking motion between each shin press.

HEALING BENEFITS

Increases blood flow to the head and neck to give your partner an alert and lively feeling.

Eases lower back pain.

12 THE HALF BRIDGE

Press your partner's knees down towards the abdomen and, with your feet slightly apart, bend your knees forwards against the arches of the feet.

Grasp the knees between your interlocked hands. Lean back with your full body weight, at the same time bending your legs to a 90° angle. Your partner's buttocks will be raised from the mat and, at the most extreme position (below), only the head, shoulders and arms will still remain on the mat. Hold for at least fifteen seconds, giving your partner's back a big stretch.

CAUTION

Don't use this technique on those with cardiac problems and high blood pressure.

13 INTIMATE BACK STRETCH

Kneeling, push your partner's legs forwards until the buttocks lift, and slide your knees and thighs under them. When you're in position, grasp your hands around the legs just above knee level and, leaning backwards, hug the legs against you to give the back a good stretch. This is a safe and gentle back stretch compared to the half bridge.

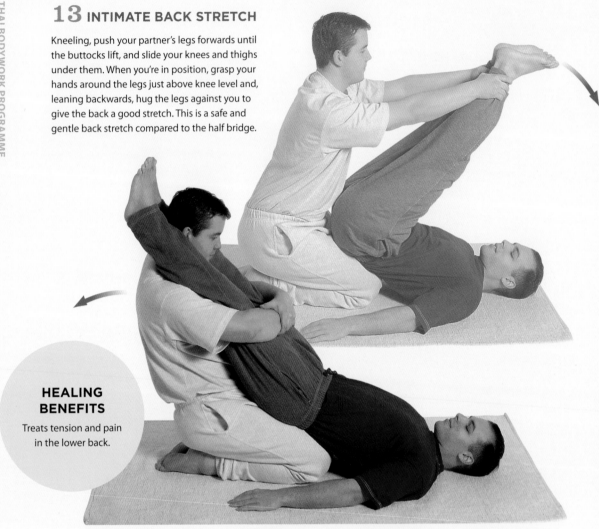

HEALING BENEFITS

Treats tension and pain in the lower back.

MUSCLES STRETCHED & PRESSED

13 Intimate back stretch
Stretched: ERECTOR SPINAE (lower back), HAMSTRINGS

14 Lifting head to straight knees
Stretched: TERES MAJOR & MINOR, BICEPS, LATISSIMUS DORSI, TRAPEZIUS, RHOMBOIDEUS, ERECTOR SPINAE, HAMSTRINGS

15 Lifting head to crossed knees
Stretched: TERES MAJOR & MINOR, RHOMBOIDEUS, BICEPS, TRAPEZIUS, ERECTOR SPINAE, GLUTEUS MAXIMUS, LATISSIMUS DORSI

14 LIFTING HEAD TO STRAIGHT KNEES

Align your partner's legs firmly against the front of your own and lean forwards to grasp each arm around the wrist. Lean your weight backwards and pull the upper body forwards and upwards.

Hold the extreme position for up to ten seconds and then gently lower your partner's upper body onto the mat. Repeat this exercise twice and maintain a slow, steady rhythm throughout.

HEALING BENEFITS
STEPS 14 & 15

Improves shoulder and hip mobility. All the stretched muscles are relaxed.

Can ease sciatic pain.

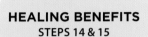

15 LIFTING HEAD TO CROSSED KNEES

As you finish the previous exercise, flex your partner's legs at the knees and cross the ankles, adjusting their position so that the side of each ankle rests against the front of your shins just below your knees. Now grasp the wrists and raise your partner's upper body towards you, just as you did in the previous technique. Hold for at least ten seconds and then repeat.

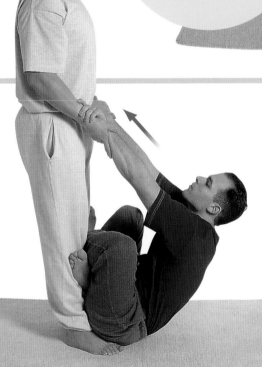

CAUTION

Good flexibility when the legs are straight isn't necessarily an accurate guide to your partner's flexibility with legs crossed. Some people have very restricted lateral movement in their hips and/or ankles but good mobility in the forwards/backwards direction.

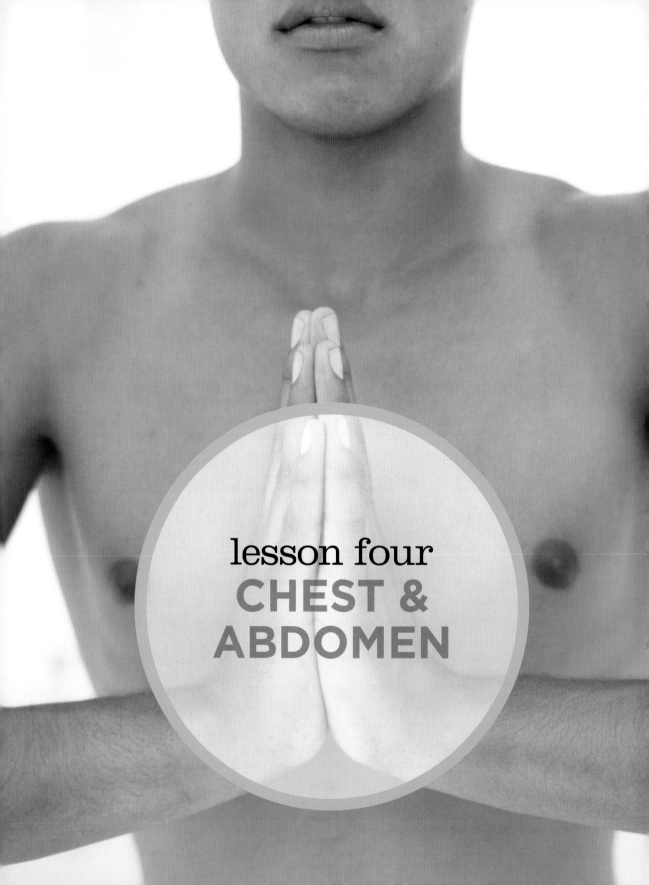

lesson four
**CHEST &
ABDOMEN**

The techniques demonstrated in Lesson Four stimulate the energies of the internal organs. Deep and thorough abdominal massage boosts the immune system. Always allow three hours after a meal before working the abdomen. Deciding on what degree of pressure is just right for a particular individual can be difficult. People vary enormously in their ability to tolerate pressure. In Western cultures, people are unused to having deep abdominal massage. Thai massage techniques for the abdomen are deeply penetrating. Be aware of your partner's facial expressions and body reactions, and always get verbal confirmation that the pressure exerted is tolerable.

SEN/MERIDIANS ON THE ABDOMEN

There are nine pressure zones on the abdomen, with the navel at the centre. Start in the lower right section and always press around the abdomen in a clockwise direction.

There are two main techniques. First, thumb walk the lines on the diagram. Start at zone **1** and thumb walk all around the edge to zone **9**. You can then vary this pattern by going **1 – 5 – 1 – 5 – 9 – 5 – 9** and then **1 – 9**.

The line that runs vertically through the belly button is the Chinese Ren Meridian.

Secondly, double palm press zones **1 – 5** on the right side and then move to the left side and press zones **6 – 9**.

These are the nine pressure points on the abdomen, which must be thoroughly pressed if energy balance in the internal organs is to be achieved.

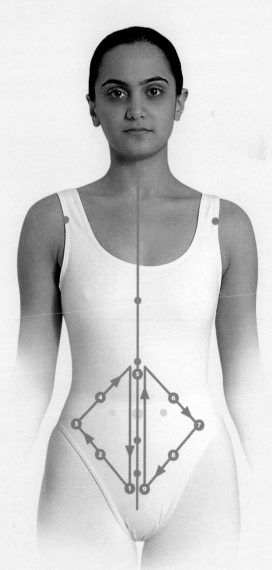

1 PRESSING THE CHEST, SHOULDERS & ARMS

With your arms straight, palm your partner's upper pectoral region using a slow, rocking movement of your body to generate pressure. If your partner is a man, you can strongly palm the entire pectoral area. Thumb knead LU 1 and R 17. Extend the palming down the arms to the hands, and back again. Repeat palming the pectorals, pressing LU 1.

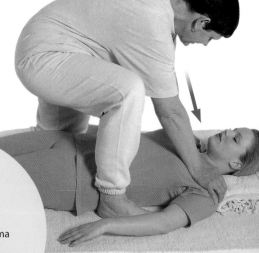

MUSCLES STRETCHED & PRESSED

1 Pressing the chest, shoulders & arms
Pressed: PECTORALS, DELTOIDS, BICEPS, WRIST EXTENSORS

3 Pressing between the ribs
Pressed: INTERCOSTALS

4 Thumb walking the abdomen
Pressed: all ABDOMINALS

5 Palm pressing the abdomen
Pressed: all ABDOMINALS

6 Pressing feet to stomach
Pressed: all ABDOMINALS

HEALING BENEFITS
STEPS 1, 2 & 3

Tonifies the lung function to benefit asthma or bronchitis sufferers.

Palming the arms contributes to the overall energy balance within the body.

2 PRESSING THE CHEST

Maintaining your position, use both hands as shown to palm press down the midline of your partner's chest on the breastbone. Press with a to and fro pushing movement to create a rocking effect and, with a female partner, always restrict your pressing to these areas.

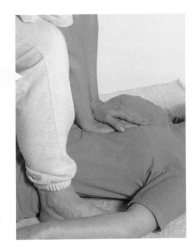

3 PRESSING BETWEEN THE RIBS (INTERCOSTAL MUSCLES)

Touch method one
Start with both thumbs either side of the sternum, just below the collarbone. Thumb press outwards along the intercostal spaces between the ribs and progress downwards. Thumb knead LU 1 and R 17. If you have a female partner, press the intercostal spaces in the centre only.

Touch method two
Use the three middle fingers of both hands to knead across the ribs with small circular movements. Again, progress downwards, observing the same precautions as above.

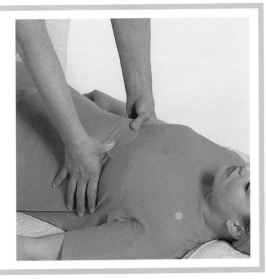

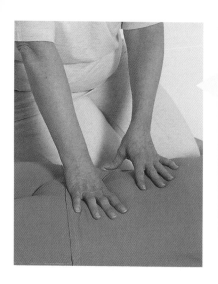

4 THUMB WALKING THE ABDOMEN

Kneeling on your partner's right, use the thumb walking technique and start just above the groin on the right side in zone 1. Thumb walk slowly, rhythmically and deeply, without causing pain, up the right side, across the abdomen just below the rib line, and down the left side to just above the pubic bone from zone 1 to zone 9.

Repeat this circuit several times and then thumb down the midline a few times. You can vary this pattern by thumbing clockwise around the two triangular areas shown on page 97. Knead ST 25, R 12, R 6 and R 4.

HEALING BENEFITS

Improves digestion and boosts internal energy.

5 PALM PRESSING THE ABDOMEN

Imagine your partner's abdomen divided into nine equal zones, with the navel in the centre. Begin in zone 1. As your partner exhales, press with the heels of both hands, aiming towards the navel, and gradually and carefully increase the pressure.

Hold for up to two minutes. Ask your partner to take a deep breath as you release the pressure. Repeat for zones 2 to 5. Move to the left and continue on zones 6 to 9.

HEALING BENEFITS
STEPS 5 & 6

Regular massage using techniques 5 and 6 aids digestion and relieves abdominal bloating and constipation.

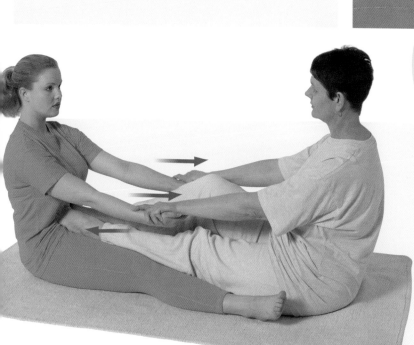

6 PRESSING FEET TO STOMACH

Sit between your partner's legs, hold hands and carefully place the balls of your feet side by side on the upper abdomen. Press alternately with care to cover the whole abdomen.

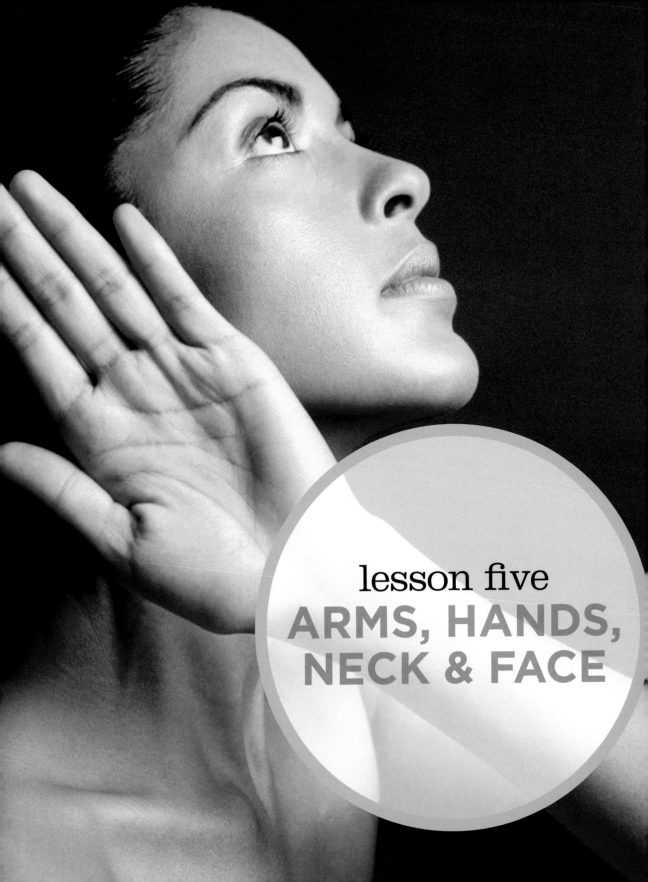

lesson five
ARMS, HANDS,
NECK & FACE

Arms feed vital energy into the body's organ systems and need thorough treatment to ensure smooth energy flow. Shoulders store tension, which causes neck pain and headaches. Stretching the shoulders and neck relieves the tension, while pressure on the head energizes and calms the mind.

SEN/MERIDIANS ON THE ARMS

INNER SEN/YIN MERIDIANS

Sen 1 Chinese Lung Meridian Runs from the lateral thumb, along the forearm to below the outer end of the clavicle (LU 1).

Sen 2 Chinese Pericardium Meridian Runs from the third finger through P 7, then through elbow and armpit to the side of the chest.

Sen 3 Chinese Heart Meridian Runs from the fifth finger, through the medial elbow HT 3, and ends in the armpit.

The inner Sen/Yin Meridians

1 Chinese Lung Meridian

2 Chinese Pericardium Meridian

3 Chinese Heart Meridian

Chinese Arm Yin Meridians start on the chest and end on the fingers. They represent the three Inner Thai Arm Sen.

OUTER SEN/YANG MERIDIANS

Sen 1 Chinese Large Intestine Meridian Starts on the index finger, runs through the wrist and the outer elbow (LI 11), up to the front of the shoulder (LI 15).

Sen 2 Chinese Sanjiao Meridian Starts on the fourth finger and passes between the radius and ulna to SJ 10 and up to the back of the arm.

Sen 3 Chinese Small Intestine Meridian Starts on the fifth finger and continues in a straight line up the back of arm to the armpit (SI 9).

The outer Sen/Meridians

1 Chinese Large Intestine Meridian

2 Chinese Sanjiao Meridian

3 Chinese Small Intestine Meridian

Chinese Leg Yang Meridians start on the hand and end on the head. They represent the three Outer Thai Arm Sen.

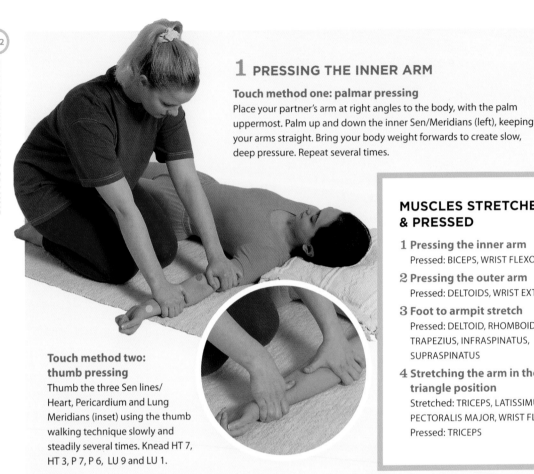

1 PRESSING THE INNER ARM

Touch method one: palmar pressing

Place your partner's arm at right angles to the body, with the palm uppermost. Palm up and down the inner Sen/Meridians (left), keeping your arms straight. Bring your body weight forwards to create slow, deep pressure. Repeat several times.

Touch method two: thumb pressing

Thumb the three Sen lines/ Heart, Pericardium and Lung Meridians (inset) using the thumb walking technique slowly and steadily several times. Knead HT 7, HT 3, P 7, P 6, LU 9 and LU 1.

MUSCLES STRETCHED & PRESSED

1 Pressing the inner arm
Pressed: BICEPS, WRIST FLEXORS

2 Pressing the outer arm
Pressed: DELTOIDS, WRIST EXTENSORS

3 Foot to armpit stretch
Pressed: DELTOID, RHOMBOIDEUS, TRAPEZIUS, INFRASPINATUS, SUPRASPINATUS

4 Stretching the arm in the triangle position
Stretched: TRICEPS, LATISSIMUS DORSI, PECTORALIS MAJOR, WRIST FLEXORS
Pressed: TRICEPS

2 PRESSING THE OUTER ARM

Touch method one

Place your partner's arm palm downwards across the chest. This exposes the outer Sen/Large Intestine, Sanjiao and Small Intestine Meridians. Palm and thumb them using the same techniques as on the inner Sen/Meridians.

Touch method two

Place your partner's arm palm downwards on the mat. Kneel behind the arm and palm and thumb the outer energy pathways again. Knead LI 11 and LI 15.

HEALING BENEFITS

Balances the body's energies. Relieves pain and stiffness in wrists, elbows and upper arms.

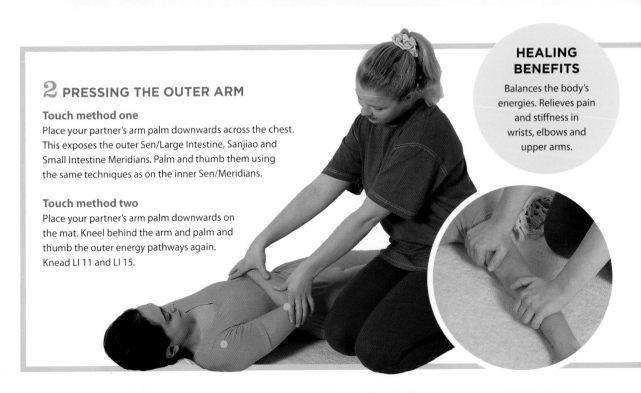

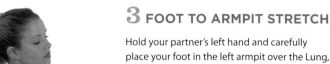

3 FOOT TO ARMPIT STRETCH

Hold your partner's left hand and carefully place your foot in the left armpit over the Lung, Pericardium and Heart Meridians. Lean back to create a strong pull against the pressure of your foot. Hold for ten seconds.

HEALING BENEFITS

Tonifies heart and lung function and stretches the arm.

CAUTION

Always ensure that the arch of your foot is placed across the actual armpit of your partner so that little pressure is exerted on the lymph nodes.

HEALING BENEFITS

Provides myofascial release for the triceps.

Improves mobility in the shoulders, elbow and wrist.

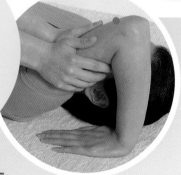

4 STRETCHING THE ARM IN THE TRIANGLE POSITION

Place the palm of your partner's left hand on the mat, with the fingers directed towards the shoulder (inset). Palm the exposed Sanjiao Meridian from elbow to armpit and back again. Knead SJ 10.

Now place your left hand on the upper thigh and your right hand on the elbow (below). Press apart with both hands to create a stretch across the trunk between arm and thigh.

5 PRESSING THE TENDONS OF THE UPPER HAND

Starting from the wrist, thumb knead along and across each of the five tendons. Knead LI 4.

HEALING BENEFITS

Strengthens the hands and eases arthritis.

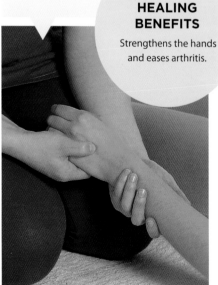

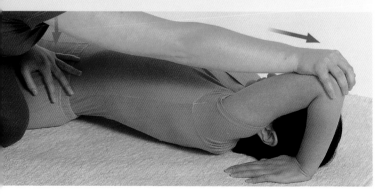

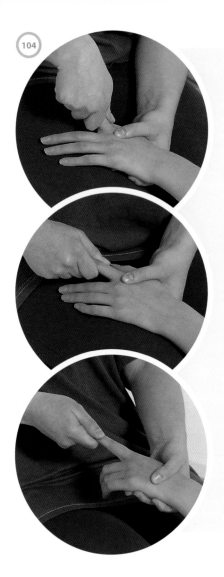

6 ROTATING, PRESSING & PULLING THE FINGERS

Touch method one
Holding each finger in turn at the fingertips, rotate the fingers several times in both directions.

Touch method two
Now squeeze up and down each finger using your index finger and thumb. Squeeze first along the top and underside of each finger, followed by lateral squeezing.

Touch method three
Pull each finger in turn and use a strong, sliding action to create a stretch. Any cracking sounds are normal and harmless. Squeeze each fingertip in turn.

HEALING BENEFITS

Strengthens the fingers and stimulates the Meridians.

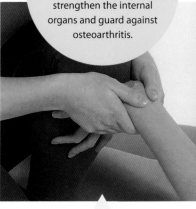

HEALING BENEFITS

Relieves carpal tunnel pain. The wrist points strengthen the internal organs and guard against osteoarthritis.

7 KNEE TO HAND PRESSING

Press your partner's left palm against your knee to strongly flex the hand backwards. Thumb press the heel of the palm and the wrist, kneading P 6, P 7, LU 9, LU 10 and HT 7.

8 INTERLOCKED HAND PRESSING

With your partner's palm uppermost, interlock your fingers with those of your partner as follows:
- The fourth finger between fingers five and four.
- Your fifth finger between fingers four and three.
- Your right-hand fifth finger between fingers three and two.
- Your third and fourth fingers between index finger and thumb.

Slide your fingers under the back of your partner's hands, leaving your thumbs free to press the inside wrist and palm. Turn your hands outwards so the sides of your partner's palms are pulled downwards, leaving them arched and stretched. Press deeply wherever you can. Knead P 8 and LU 10.

HEALING BENEFITS

Stretches the palm to free fibrotic tissue. P 8 calms and LU 10 eases thumb pain.

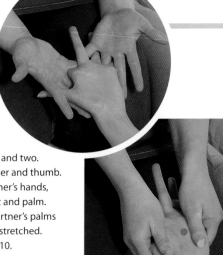

MUSCLES STRETCHED & PRESSED

7 Knee to hand pressing
  Stretched: HAND FLEXORS

8 Interlocked hand pressing
  Stretched: HAND FLEXORS

9 Rotating the wrist
  Stretched: WRIST & HAND
  FLEXORS & EXTENSORS

10 Pulling the arms
  Stretched: TRAPEZIUS, DELTOIDS,
  INFRASPINATUS, RHOMBOIDEUS,
  BICEPS, PECTORALIS MAJOR

9 ROTATING THE WRIST

Support your partner's forearm near the wrist and use an interlocked finger grip to rotate the wrist strongly, first one way and then the other.

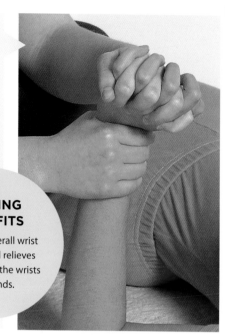

HEALING BENEFITS

Improves overall wrist mobility and relieves numbness of the wrists and hands.

10 PULLING THE ARMS

Touch method one: vertical arms
Standing behind your partner's shoulders, grasp both hands and then pull both arms up and down, lifting each shoulder alternately.

HEALING BENEFITS

Reduces tension in the shoulders and improves mobility.

Stimulates the six arm Meridians.

Touch method two: backwards pull
Now step back from your partner and pull both arms together, leaning with your body weight to create the pull.

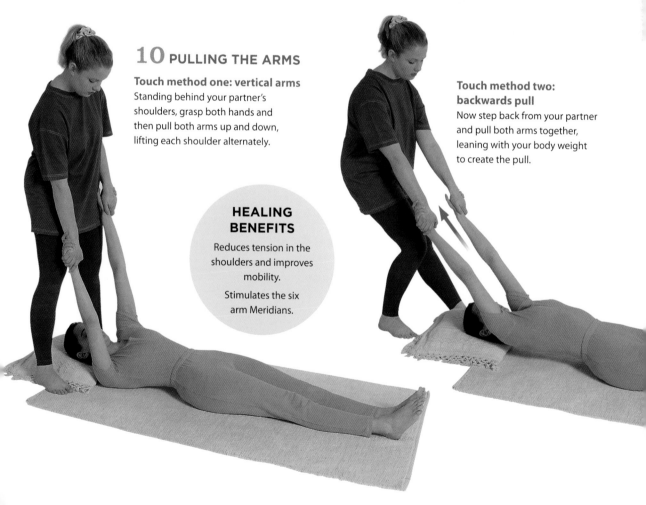

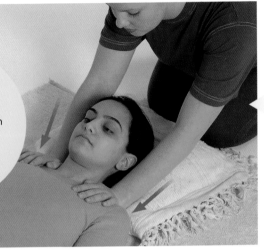

HEALING BENEFITS

GB 21 removes tension from the neck and shoulders, and LU 1 tonifies the lungs.

11 PRESSING THE SHOULDERS

Kneel behind your partner's head. Press the top of the shoulders with both hands to stretch the muscles. Then press alternately with a gentle, rocking motion. Thumb knead GB 21. Finally, thumb press along the collarbone and over the upper pectoral muscles. Knead LU 1.

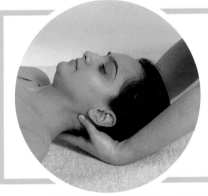

12 PRESSING THE NECK

Support the base of your partner's head with one hand, lifting it slightly so that, with the other hand, you can thumb up and down the neck muscles on the Gall Bladder and Bladder Meridians. Knead GB 20 and BL 10.

Turn the head gently to one side and thumb knead along the sternocleidomastoid muscle. Swap hands and repeat on the other side.

13 STRETCHING THE NECK

Place both hands under your partner's lower neck and pull them towards you to create a mild traction on the neck. Repeat several times. Keeping a slight traction, press with your fingers into the soft tissue immediately behind the base of the skull. Hold for up to one minute. Allow the weight of the head to generate the pressure.

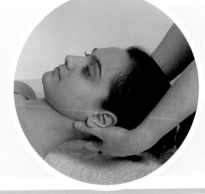

HEALING BENEFITS

Relaxes the neck muscles, eases headaches and improves mobility of the neck.

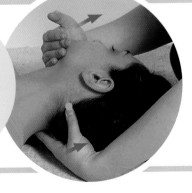

14 PULLING THE TURNED HEAD

Place your right hand under your partner's chin and your left hand under the base of the skull, using equal pressure with both hands. Pull the head back very gently and carefully. Hold the pull for at least ten seconds.

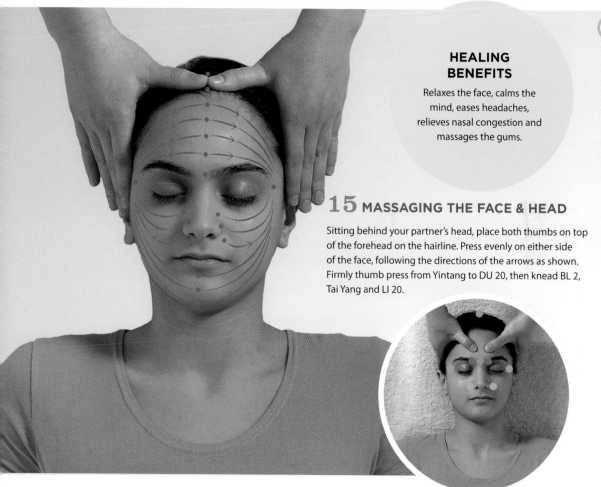

15 MASSAGING THE FACE & HEAD

Sitting behind your partner's head, place both thumbs on top of the forehead on the hairline. Press evenly on either side of the face, following the directions of the arrows as shown. Firmly thumb press from Yintang to DU 20, then knead BL 2, Tai Yang and LI 20.

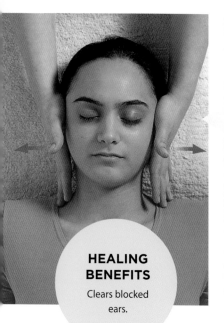

16 MASSAGING THE EARS

Cup and cover your partner's ears with the palm of your hands to create a suction. Hold for thirty seconds and then release.

MUSCLES STRETCHED & PRESSED

11 **Pressing the shoulders**
   Pressed: TRAPEZIUS

12 **Pressing the neck**
   Pressed: STERNOCLEIDOMASTOID, LEVATOR SCAPULAE

14 **Pulling the turned head**
   Stretched: STERNOCLEIDOMASTOID, TRAPEZIUS, ERECTOR SPINAE, LEVATOR SCAPULAE

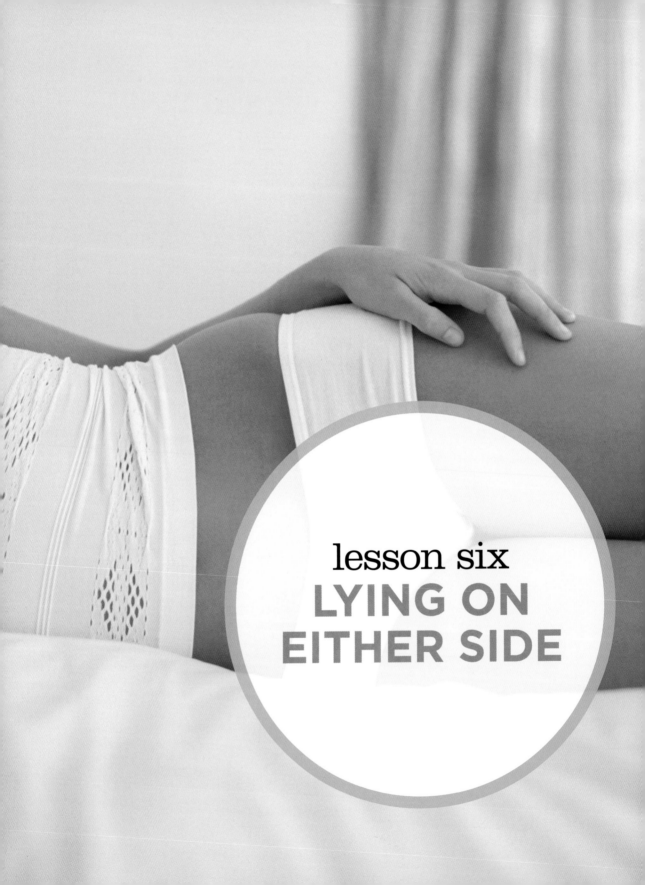

lesson six
LYING ON
EITHER SIDE

The techniques featured in this lesson give access to the Sen/Meridians in the side position and provide an opportunity to reach muscles that can't be treated effectively in the other positions. Each side of the body is treated in turn, first with your partner on one side using techniques 1–23, which are then repeated when lying on the other side. If you decide to do only some of the techniques shown, remember to repeat each one on the other side of the body. Refer to chapter 2 (see pages 42–51) for the basic techniques of pressing and manipulation.

SEN/MERIDIANS IN THE SIDE POSITION

The Sen/Meridians in the legs and back are described and illustrated anatomically in Lessons Two and Seven (see pages 64 and 122). In the side position, the bent leg exposes **Sen 2** – Chinese Gallbladder Meridian, which treats side hip and leg pain, and **Sen 3** – Chinese Bladder Meridian, which energetically influences the internal organs of the body and strengthens the back.

The back of the straight leg also exposes **Sen 3** – Chinese Bladder Meridian.

There's only one Sen line on each side of the spine. The Chinese Bladder Meridian has two lines.

— **Sen 2**
— **Sen 3**

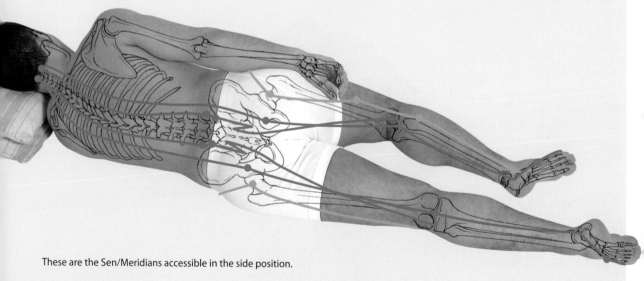

These are the Sen/Meridians accessible in the side position.

1 PRESSING THE BACK OF THE EXTENDED LEG

Touch method one: palmar pressing (below) Place your partner's right leg at 90° to the body. Keeping your arms straight, palm with both hands along the inner Sen/Kidney, Spleen and Liver Meridians of the straight leg, using your body weight to generate deep pressure. Palm outwards from the knee and back again several times. Keep a steady rhythm using a slow, to and fro rocking movement. Then butterfly palm the entire leg.

HEALING BENEFITS

Pressing the inner Sen/ Meridians promotes efficient abdominal organ functions and prevents swollen legs.

Touch method two: thumb walking (inset) Starting on your partner's inside lower leg, thumb walk deeply along the energy pathways. Press-knead K 3, SP 6 and SP 9.

2 PRESSING THE FLEXED LEG

Palm the outer Sen 3/ Gall Bladder Meridian of your partner's flexed leg. Then thumb walk it up and down on the lower leg and the upper leg in turn. Knead GB 31, GB 34, GB 40 and ST 36.

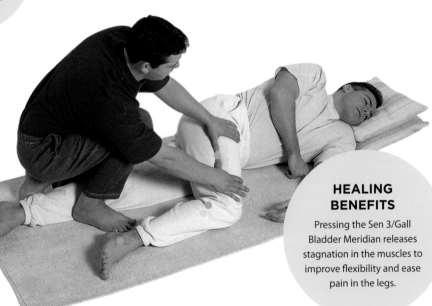

HEALING BENEFITS

Pressing the Sen 3/Gall Bladder Meridian releases stagnation in the muscles to improve flexibility and ease pain in the legs.

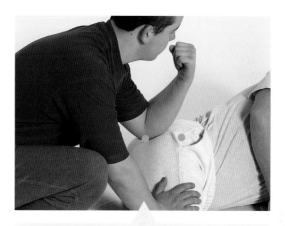

MUSCLES STRETCHED & PRESSED

1 Pressing the back of the extended leg
Pressed: SOLEUS, GASTROCNEMIUS, HAMSTRINGS, ADDUCTOR MUSCLE

2 Pressing the flexed leg
Pressed: GLUTEUS MAXIMUS, BICEPS FEMORIS, TENSOR FASCIAE LATAE, VASTUS LATERALIS, ILIOTIBIAL TRACT

3 Pressing around the hip joint
Pressed: GLUTEUS MAXIMUS, BICEPS FEMORIS, RECTUS FEMORIS, TENSOR FASCIAE LATAE

4 Side single grape press
Pressed: HAMSTRINGS, GLUTEUS MAXIMUS, ADDUCTORS, GRACILIS

3 PRESSING AROUND THE HIP JOINT

With your partner's right leg still in the flexed position, press deeply with your thumbs and palms around the hip joint. Finally, elbow press GB 30, GB 29 and BL 54 by leaning in gradually with your body weight to give more pressure.

HEALING BENEFITS

Wonderfully effective in the treatment of sciatica and hip pain.

4 SIDE SINGLE GRAPE PRESS

Grasp both your partner's ankles and use your right foot to press up and down the thigh on Sen 3/ Bladder Meridian. Generate pressure by leaning back and pulling both legs.

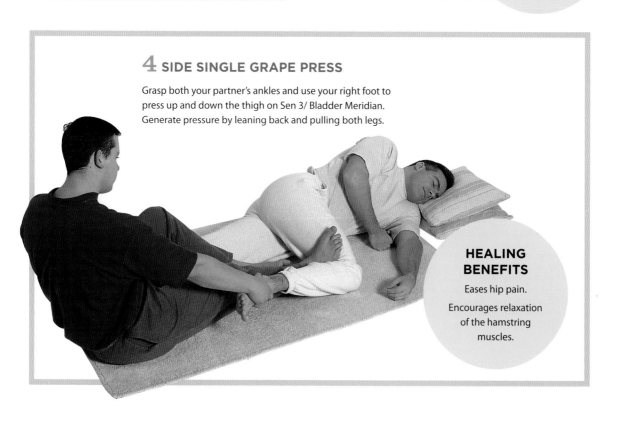

HEALING BENEFITS

Eases hip pain.

Encourages relaxation of the hamstring muscles.

5 SIDE SINGLE GRAPE PRESS & TWISTED VINE

As you complete the previous technique, tuck your foot behind your partner's right knee and cross the right foot over your right shin. Tuck the toes in behind your knee, holding the heel with your right hand. Press up and down your partner's thigh using your left foot.

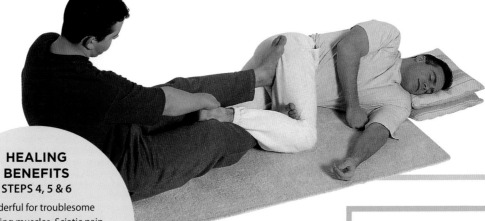

HEALING BENEFITS
STEPS 4, 5 & 6

Wonderful for troublesome hamstring muscles. Sciatic pain felt deeply within the leg also responds well to these treatments.

Leaves the leg suffused with warmth and feeling really light.

6 SIDE Z-STOP

Follow exactly the same method as used for this technique in the supine position (see page 72).

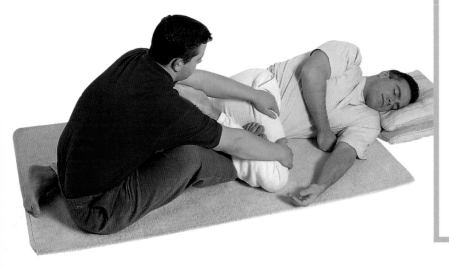

MUSCLES STRETCHED & PRESSED

5 Side single grape press & twisted vine
Pressed: HAMSTRINGS, GLUTEUS MAXIMUS, ADDUCTORS, GRACILIS

6 Side z-stop
Stretched: QUADRICEPS
Pressed: HAMSTRINGS, QUADRICEPS

7 Foot pressing thighs & calves with chair
Pressed: GASTROCNEMIUS, SOLEUS, HAMSTRINGS

8 Pressing the back in the side position
Pressed: ERECTOR SPINAE, LATISSIMUS DORSI, GLUTEUS MAXIMUS, QUADRATUS LUMBORUM, TRAPEZIUS, INFRASPINATUS, RHOMBOIDEUS MAJOR & MINOR

CAUTION

Don't attempt this exercise on someone who is lighter than you.

7 FOOT PRESSING THIGHS & CALVES WITH CHAIR

Use a chair to provide you with support as you very carefully step onto the lower part of your partner's flexed legs only, as shown. Without moving the position of your feet on the legs, slowly rock from one foot to the other. Now move your feet to a new position and then repeat.

HEALING BENEFITS

Relaxes tense and sore muscles and tendons; eases sciatic pain.

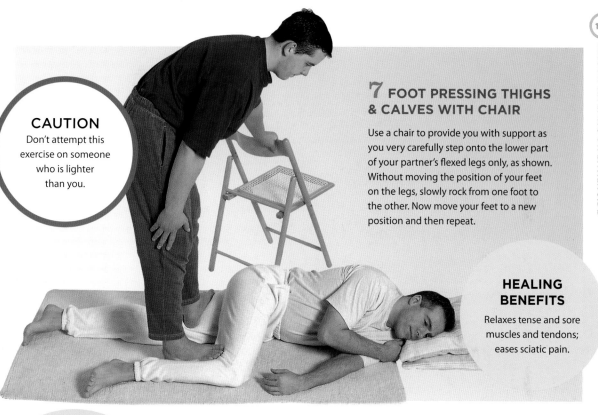

HEALING BENEFITS

Pushes the muscles away from the spine, relieving back pain and tension. Stimulates energy flow in the internal organs.

8 PRESSING THE BACK IN THE SIDE POSITION

Touch method one: palmar pressing (below)
Kneel behind your partner and make sure that the left leg is flexed in front to give good support when pressure is applied to the back. Palm press along the Sen/Bladder Meridian on the left of the spine with a rocking movement.

Touch method two: thumb pressing (inset) Thumb walk sideways along the same lines on your partner's back. Knead BL 25 and BL 26.

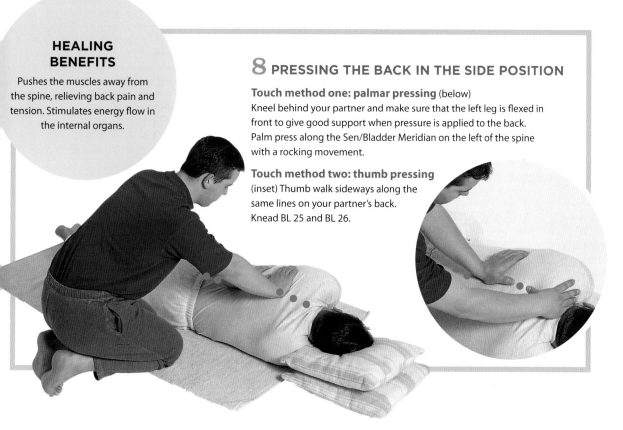

9 ROTATING THE SHOULDER

Grasp your partner's right shoulder firmly with
both your hands. Rotate the shoulder according to
its flexibility through its full range of movement.
Knead GB 20. Press into GB 21 and stretch
backwards. Knead GB 20. Knead LI 15 and SJ 14.

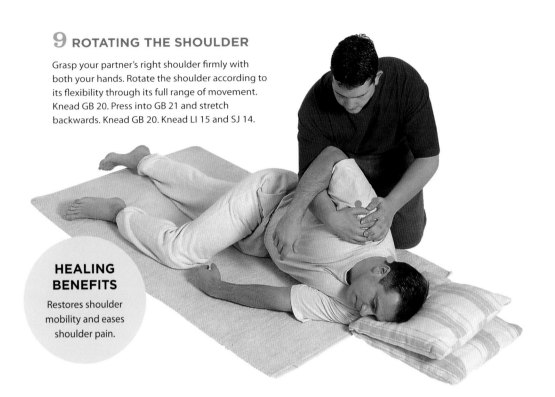

HEALING BENEFITS

Restores shoulder
mobility and eases
shoulder pain.

10 ROTATING THE SHOULDER WITH ELBOW LEVER

Maintain your grasp on your partner's right shoulder and place
your right elbow on the lower back to the right of the spine on
BL 25. Lean forwards so that you can use your elbow as a lever
against which you can pull the shoulder as you rotate.

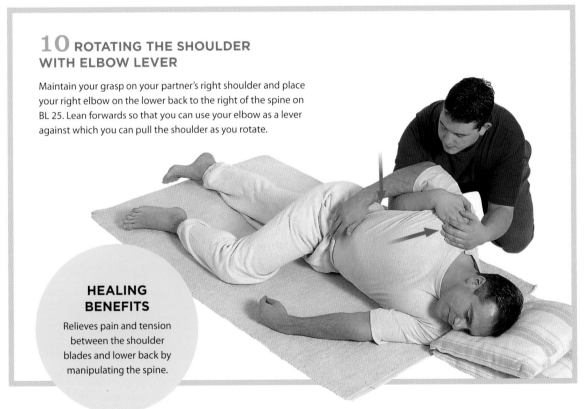

HEALING BENEFITS

Relieves pain and tension
between the shoulder
blades and lower back by
manipulating the spine.

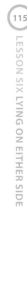

11 PRESSING THE KNEE-SUPPORTED ARM

Extend your partner's right arm and lay it across your left knee.
Then palm up and down the arm slowly and firmly several times on the
Sen 1/Lung Meridian and Sen 2/Pericardium Meridian. Press under the
collarbone on LU 1 while stretching the arm back.

HEALING BENEFITS

Stretches the pectoral
muscles and assists
myofascial release in
the deltoid and
biceps muscles.

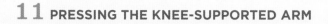

MUSCLES STRETCHED & PRESSED

9 Rotating the shoulder
Stretched: UPPER TRAPEZIUS,
PECTORALIS MAJOR, INFRASPINATUS,
RHOMBOIDEUS MINOR & MAJOR

**10 Rotating the shoulder
with elbow lever**
Stretched: PECTORALIS MAJOR,
TRAPEZIUS, STERNOCLEIDOMASTOID,
LEVATOR SCAPULAE

**11 Pressing the
knee-supported arm**
Pressed: BICEPS, DELTOID, FLEXOR
MUSCLES OF THE WRISTS & HANDS

**12 Stretching the vertical
arm sideways**
Stretched: PECTORALIS MAJOR,
TRAPEZIUS, RHOMBOIDEUS,
TERES MAJOR, INFRASPINATUS

12 STRETCHING THE VERTICAL ARM SIDEWAYS

Holding your partner's right hand and wrist, tuck the
outside of your lower right leg snugly against your
partner's back across the shoulder blades. As you lean
back, pull vertically upwards and backwards on the
arm, which will be stretched against the outer margin
of your right leg. Hold the extreme position for a few
seconds and then relax. Repeat several times.

HEALING BENEFITS

Improves shoulder
mobility.

Eases tension and pain
in the elbow region.

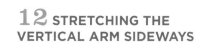

MUSCLES STRETCHED & PRESSED

13 Pulling the arm in the side position
Stretched: LATISSIMUS DORSI, TERES MAJOR, SUBSCAPULARIS

14 Pressing the arm against the side
Pressed: DELTOID, BICEPS, TRICEPS, HAND & WRIST EXTENSORS

15 Stretching the arm in the triangle position
Stretched: LATISSIMUS DORSI, TRICEPS, PECTORALIS MAJOR, HAND & WRIST FLEXORS, ABDOMINAL OBLIQUES, QUADRATUS LUMBORUM, TERES MAJOR

16 Shoulder to opposite knee spinal twist
Stretched: ABDOMINAL OBLIQUES, QUADRATUS LUMBORUM, GLUTEUS MAXIMUS, PECTORALIS MAJOR
Pressed: PECTORALIS MAJOR, VASTUS LATERALIS, QUADRICEPS

HEALING BENEFITS

Opens up the shoulder and elbow joints and stimulates the circulation of blood and lymph.

Aids and maintains joint mobility, which is especially beneficial for frozen shoulders and tennis elbow.

13 PULLING THE ARM IN THE SIDE POSITION

Change your position to pull your partner's arm right back over the head. Relax and then repeat this technique two or three times, holding the extreme position in each instance for a few seconds.

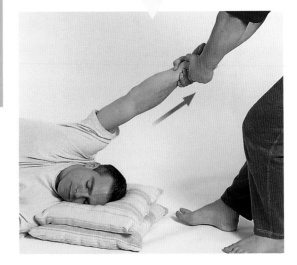

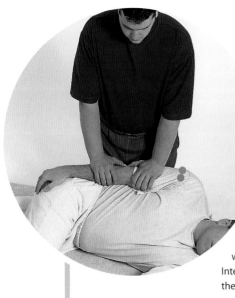

14 PRESSING THE ARM AGAINST THE SIDE

Lay the right arm along the side of the body. Press and then thumb walk with both hands along the outer Sen/Large Intestine, Sanjiao and Small Intestine Meridians of the arm (see page 101). Knead LI 15, SJ 14, SJ 10 and LI 11. Press the wrist and shoulder outwards to give the arm a stretch.

HEALING BENEFITS

Stimulates the flow of energy pathways, which contributes to overall energy balance.

15 STRETCHING THE ARM IN THE TRIANGLE POSITION

Flex your partner's arm at the elbow and place the hand behind the head with fingers directed towards the shoulder. Palm the exposed upper arm and along the side of the body to the hips. Carefully, stretch the side, pressing SJ 10 on the elbow and GB 29 on the hip.

HEALING BENEFITS

Stretches muscles down the side of the body that rarely experience any strong extension.

16 SHOULDER TO OPPOSITE KNEE SPINAL TWIST

With your left hand on your partner's right shoulder and your other hand on the right knee, press down and outwards carefully to generate a good stretch, with a twisting action on the spine. Hold the twist for a few seconds.

HEALING BENEFITS

Aids spinal flexibility and eases back pain.

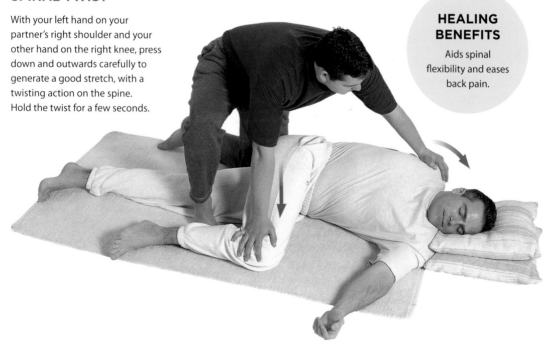

17 KNEE TO KNEE HIP FLEX

Step over your partner's left leg and press your left leg tightly against it. Hold the right ankle and tuck your right knee behind your partner's while you press down on the right hip. Then push forwards and rock with your knee to generate a series of strong hip flexions.

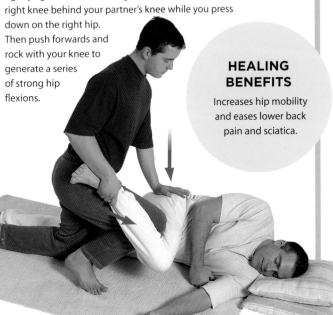

HEALING BENEFITS

Increases hip mobility and eases lower back pain and sciatica.

MUSCLES STRETCHED & PRESSED

17 Knee to knee hip flex
Stretched: GLUTEUS MAXIMUS, RECTUS FEMORIS
Pressed: HAMSTRINGS, GLUTEUS MAXIMUS

18 Stretching the crossed leg horizontally
Stretched: GLUTEUS MAXIMUS, PIRIFORMIS, HAMSTRINGS, GASTROCNEMIUS, SOLEUS
Pressed: GLUTEUS MAXIMUS, TENSOR FASCIAE LATAE

19 Knee pivot hip stretch
Stretched: QUADRICEPS, GRACILIS, SARTORIUS, ADDUCTORS, ILIACUS, PSOAS MAJOR
Pressed: GLUTEUS MAXIMUS

20 Side back bow
Stretched: QUADRICEPS, PSOAS MAJOR, ILIACUS, RECTUS ABDOMINIS, PECTORALIS MAJOR
Pressed: ERECTOR SPINAE, GLUTEUS MAXIMUS

HEALING BENEFITS

Improves hip flexibility and eases sciatica and tension in the buttocks, lower back and hamstrings.

18 STRETCHING THE CROSSED LEG HORIZONTALLY

Stretch the right leg across the left hip, holding the right ankle and pressing down onto GB 29 on the right hip. With your knee pressing into the Sen/Bladder Meridian, carefully stretch the straight leg by pushing towards your partner's head.

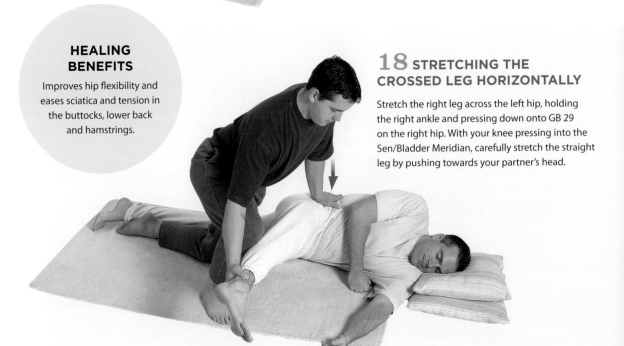

19 KNEE PIVOT HIP STRETCH

Place your left knee in the centre of your partner's right
buttock on GB 30. Grasp the right leg and pull it towards
you, using your knee as a pivot to help generate a big
stretch in the muscles at the front of the hip and thigh.
Hold for 60 seconds, and repeat several times.

HEALING BENEFITS

GB 30 is a major
point for easing hip
pain and sciatica.

20 SIDE BACK BOW

Seat yourself on the floor behind your partner, with your legs
outstretched. Position your feet so that the right one is against
the pelvic arch and the left one is across the lumbar region.

Pull your partner's arm and leg towards you, leaning
backwards to pull the back against your feet, so creating
a bow shape through the arm, spine and leg. Hold this pose
for a minute or more.

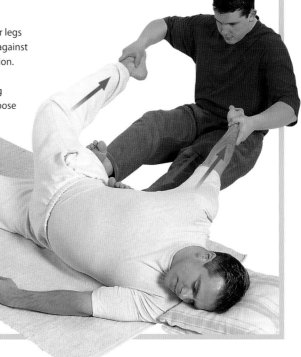

HEALING BENEFITS

Improves flexibility of
the spine in a backwards
direction and eases lower
back pain.

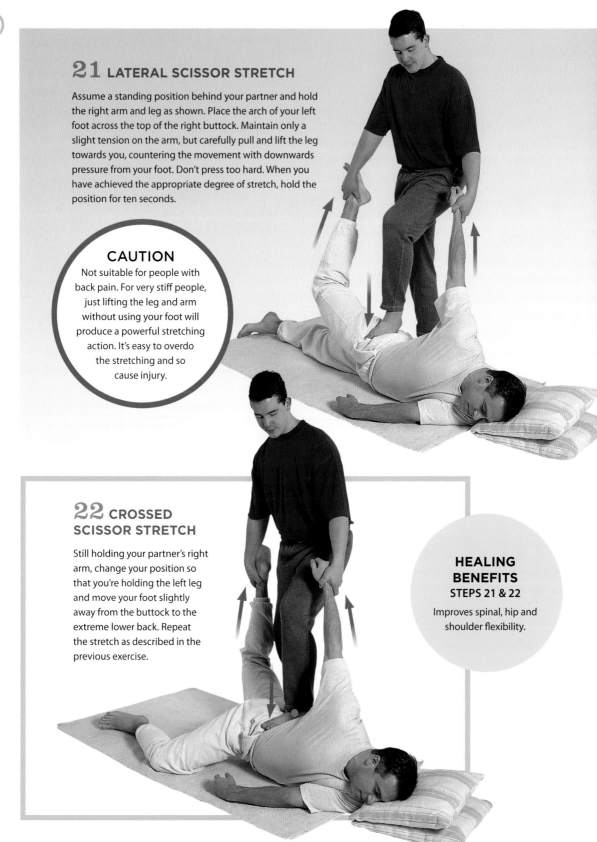

21 LATERAL SCISSOR STRETCH

Assume a standing position behind your partner and hold the right arm and leg as shown. Place the arch of your left foot across the top of the right buttock. Maintain only a slight tension on the arm, but carefully pull and lift the leg towards you, countering the movement with downwards pressure from your foot. Don't press too hard. When you have achieved the appropriate degree of stretch, hold the position for ten seconds.

CAUTION

Not suitable for people with back pain. For very stiff people, just lifting the leg and arm without using your foot will produce a powerful stretching action. It's easy to overdo the stretching and so cause injury.

22 CROSSED SCISSOR STRETCH

Still holding your partner's right arm, change your position so that you're holding the left leg and move your foot slightly away from the buttock to the extreme lower back. Repeat the stretch as described in the previous exercise.

HEALING BENEFITS
STEPS 21 & 22

Improves spinal, hip and shoulder flexibility.

MUSCLES STRETCHED & PRESSED

21 Lateral scissor stretch
Stretched: RECTUS ABDOMINIS, ILIACUS, PSOAS MAJOR, ADDUCTORS, PECTORALIS MAJOR, SARTORIUS
Pressed: VASTUS LATERALIS

22 Crossed scissor stretch
Stretched: as lateral scissor stretch
Pressed: VASTUS LATERALIS

23 Pulling spinal twist
Stretched: QUADRATUS LUMBORUM, TRAPEZIUS, TERES MAJOR, ERECTOR SPINAE, DELTOID, RHOMBOIDEUS MINOR & MAJOR, INFRASPINATUS, SUBCAPULARIS
Pressed: GLUTEUS MAXIMUS

24 Lifting spinal twist
Stretched: QUADRATUS LUMBORUM, TRAPEZIUS, TERES MAJOR, ERECTOR SPINAE, RHOMBOIDEUS MAJOR & MINOR, INFRASPINATUS, SUBCAPULARIS

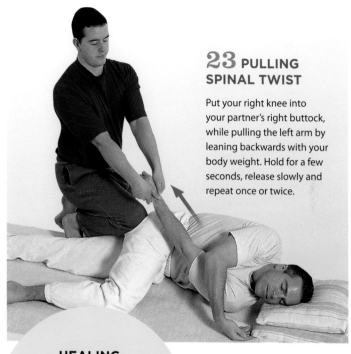

23 PULLING SPINAL TWIST

Put your right knee into your partner's right buttock, while pulling the left arm by leaning backwards with your body weight. Hold for a few seconds, release slowly and repeat once or twice.

HEALING BENEFITS
STEPS 23 & 24

Stretches the Small Intestine Meridian to ease frozen shoulder and muscle pain between the scapulae.

24 LIFTING SPINAL TWIST

Bend your partner's right leg to form a 90° angle in front. Tuck your right foot under the flexed knee and place your left foot on the mat so that the inner margin of your lower leg is firmly against your partner's lower back.

Hold the left wrist as shown and lean backwards using your weight to lift the body. Hold for several seconds before lowering your partner gently to the floor. Repeat twice.

CAUTION

Don't practise this exercise on anyone who has had spinal surgery such as lumbar fusion or laminectomy, those with osteoporosis or anyone who's much heavier than yourself.

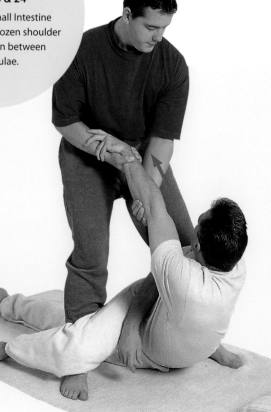

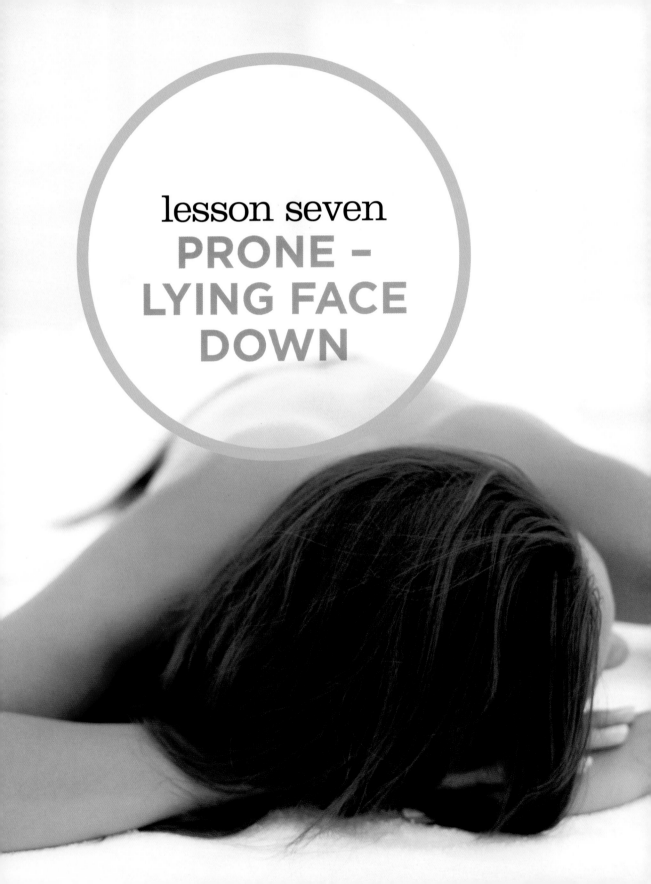

lesson seven
PRONE - LYING FACE DOWN

The ultimate energy balance throughout the body can only be achieved by pressing the Sen/Bladder Meridian on either side of the spine. Energy flow in this area affects all the organ systems and the overall health and well-being of the body. The powerful manipulations demonstrated in this lesson will strengthen the spine and help to treat all kinds of back problems.

Refer to chapter 2 (see pages 42–51) for the basic techniques of pressing and manipulation. Energy flow through the legs and hips relaxes muscle and improves mobility in the lower back as well as all leg and hip joints.

SEN/MERIDIAN ON THE BACK

There's only one Sen line on each side of the spine. The Chinese Bladder Meridian, however, has two lines – the inner one is two finger-widths and the outer one four finger-widths from the midline of the spine.

The Bladder Meridian starts on the eye and ends on the outer edge of the little toe in one continuous energy pathway. In Thai bodywork, pressing is done from the feet up to the buttocks. The back Sen/Bladder Meridian starts between the ankle bone and the Achilles tendon and then runs up the midline of the back of the leg.

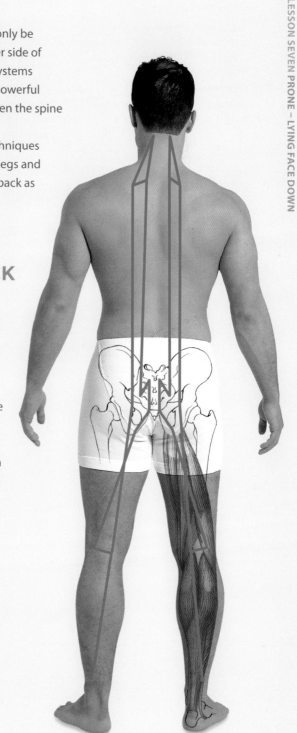

The Chinese Bladder Meridian, representing the Thai back Sen, runs the full length of the spine on both sides. Focused pressure on it enhances general health and flexibility.

1 STANDING FEET TO FEET PRESS

Balancing your weight on your toes, lean backwards to press your heels into K 1 and around the soles of your partner's feet. Use a gentle to and fro rocking motion with your feet.

NOTE: make sure you have adequate padding beneath your partner's feet for this exercise.

HEALING BENEFITS

Improves blood flow as the metatarsal bones are splayed apart. K 1 strengthens the spine.

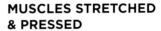

MUSCLES STRETCHED & PRESSED

1 Standing feet to feet press
Pressed: all intrinsic muscles of the feet

2 Pressing the back of the legs & buttocks
Pressed: GASTROCNEMIUS, SOLEUS, HAMSTRINGS

3 Pressing heel to buttock
Stretched: TIBIALIS ANTERIOR, QUADRICEPS, FOOT FLEXORS

4 Pressing the thigh & pulling the foot
Stretched: TIBIALIS ANTERIOR, FOOT FLEXORS
Pressed: HAMSTRINGS

5 Foot cracker
Stretched: TIBIALIS ANTERIOR, QUADRICEPS, FOOT FLEXORS
Pressed: HAMSTRINGS, GASTROCNEMIUS

2 PRESSING THE BACK OF THE LEGS & BUTTOCKS

Touch method one: palmar and thumb pressing

Assume a kneeling position and palmar press several times up both legs from the ankles to the lower margin of the buttocks. Thumb press up the centre Sen 3/Bladder Meridian of the legs, kneading BL 57, BL 40, BL 37 and BL 36 (see page 65). Repeat several times.

Touch method two: butterfly pressing

Butterfly press up each leg in turn several times.

CAUTION

Don't use the deep palming or thumbing method on areas with obvious varicose veins.

HEALING BENEFITS

Pressing the Bladder Meridian releases myofascial adhesions to prevent and treat lower back pain.

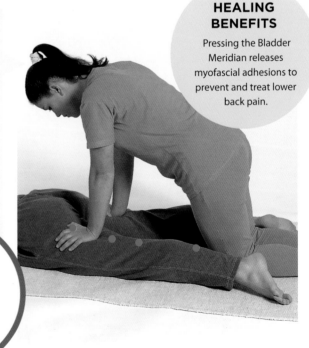

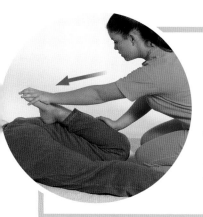

3 PRESSING HEEL TO BUTTOCK

Press your partner's right foot back as far towards the buttocks as is comfortable. At the same time, use the heel of your right palm to press along the Sen 1/Stomach Meridian, which lies just outside the margin of the tibia – see page 65.

HEALING BENEFITS

Stretches quadriceps to release tension, and improves ankle and knee mobility.

4 PRESSING THE THIGH & PULLING THE FOOT

Grasp your partner's foot with both hands and place your right foot across the back of the thigh on Sen 3/Bladder Meridian, close to the knee crease. Pull the lower leg vertically upwards and hold for a few seconds. Repeat progressively up the thigh, focusing on BL 37.

HEALING BENEFITS

Eases sciatic pain and relieves pain and tension in the hamstring muscles. Aids ankle flexibility and stimulates the energy pathways.

5 FOOT CRACKER

Still standing, tuck your left foot in snugly behind your partner's right knee and press the foot down towards the buttock.

HEALING BENEFITS

Improves mobility of the ankle and knee joints; eases tension and spasming in calves and hamstrings.

HEALING BENEFITS

Eases lower back and hip pain, and sciatica.

6 STANDING BACKWARDS LEG LIFT

Facing your partner's feet, grasp the right ankle and then lift the leg backwards as far as is comfortable.

Now repeat techniques 3–6 on the other leg.

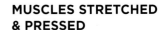

MUSCLES STRETCHED & PRESSED

6 Standing backwards leg lift
Stretched: ILIACUS, PSOAS MAJOR, QUADRICEPS, SARTORIUS

7 Pressing feet to buttock
Stretched: ANTERIOR TIBIALIS, QUADRICEPS, FOOT FLEXORS, SOLEUS

8 Reverse half lotus press
Pressed: HAMSTRINGS, VASTUS LATERALIS, GASTROCNEMIUS, PERONEUS LONGUS

9 Reverse half lotus leg flex
Stretched: TIBIALIS ANTERIOR, QUADRICEPS, PSOAS MAJOR, ADDUCTORS, SARTORIUS
Pressed: HAMSTRINGS, VASTUS LATERALIS

10 Reverse half lotus leg lift
Stretched: PSOAS MAJOR, QUADRICEPS, ILIACUS
Pressed: SACROSPINALIS

HEALING BENEFITS

Increases mobility of the feet, ankles and knees.

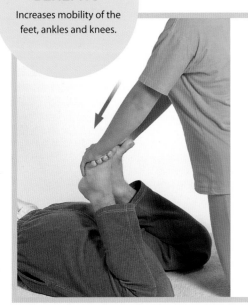

7 PRESSING FEET TO BUTTOCK

Touch method one (left)
Press both your partner's feet down towards the buttocks and simultaneously pull down on the balls of the feet.

Touch method two (right)
Cross your partner's legs and press both feet down to the buttocks. Recross the legs in the opposite way and then repeat.

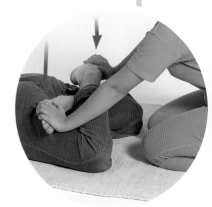

8 REVERSE HALF LOTUS PRESS

Bend your partner's right leg into the half lotus position so that the top of the foot lies across the left thigh just behind the knee crease. Now palm and thumb walk along the outer Sen 2/Gall Bladder Meridian of the flexed leg (see page 65). Knead GB 30.

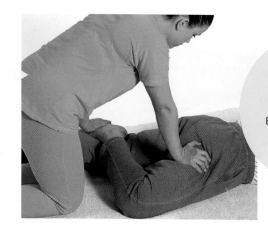

HEALING BENEFITS

Eases pain and tension in the hip and thighs.

HEALING BENEFITS

Improves flexibility in the hip and knee joints. Treats chronic pain in the iliosacral region.

9 REVERSE HALF LOTUS LEG FLEX

From the same half lotus position, grasp your partner's left foot, as shown, and push it down towards the buttock. Then with each push forwards simultaneously press the other thigh.

10 REVERSE HALF LOTUS LEG LIFT

Retaining the half lotus position of the legs, grasp your partner's left foot with both hands and stand up. Place your right foot carefully across the lower lumbar area on BL 25 and BL 26, without using your full body weight as you lift the leg.

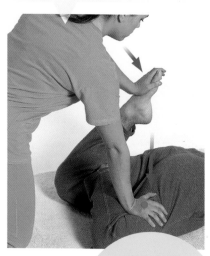

CAUTION

Only with a highly flexible partner will you be able to lift the leg to anywhere near the vertical position.

HEALING BENEFITS

Stimulates blood flow and lymphatic drainage, and treats painful and spasming hamstrings and sciatica.

HEALING BENEFITS

Helps those who suffer from lumbar pain, hip pain and sciatica.

11 KNEE OR HAND TO BUTTOCK/BACK LEG LIFT

Touch method one (below)
Place your right knee into your partner's right buttock (BL 54 or GB 30) and lift the leg with your left hand under the knee, using your knee as the pivot and your right hand for support.

Touch method two (inset)
With the heel of your right hand pressing into the right BL 25 and BL 26, lift the right flexed leg against the pressure of your hand.

HEALING BENEFITS
STEPS 12 & 13

Eases tension and pain in front of the thigh, and helps sciatica and lower back pain.

12 FOOT TO BUTTOCK/BACK BACKWARDS LEG LIFT

Hold your partner's right foot with both hands and lift the leg. Now place your left foot across the lower lumbar area and lean back to pull the leg against pressure from the foot.

MUSCLES STRETCHED & PRESSED

11 Knee or hand to buttock/back leg lift
Stretched: GRACILIS, QUADRICEPS
Pressed: GLUTEUS MAXIMUS

12 Foot to buttock/back backwards leg lift
Stretched: ILIACUS, PSOAS MAJOR, QUADRICEPS
Pressed: GLUTEUS MAXIMUS, SACROSPINALIS

13 Backwards seesaw leg lift
Stretched: PSOAS MAJOR, ILIACUS, QUADRICEPS, SARTORIUS
Pressed: GLUTEUS MAXIMUS

14 Intimate calf & thigh press
Stretched: GLUTEUS, BICEPS FEMORIS, VASTUS LATERALIS
Pressed: GLUTEUS, BICEPS FEMORIS, VASTUS LATERALIS

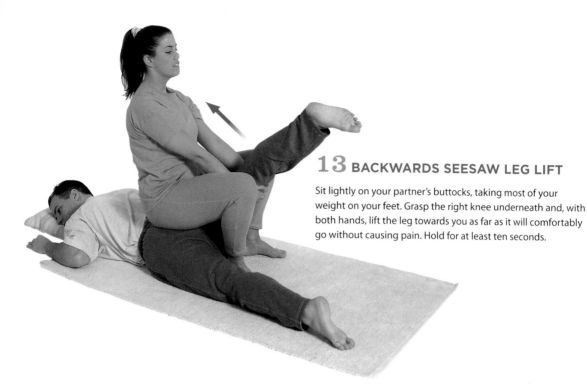

13 BACKWARDS SEESAW LEG LIFT

Sit lightly on your partner's buttocks, taking most of your weight on your feet. Grasp the right knee underneath and, with both hands, lift the leg towards you as far as it will comfortably go without causing pain. Hold for at least ten seconds.

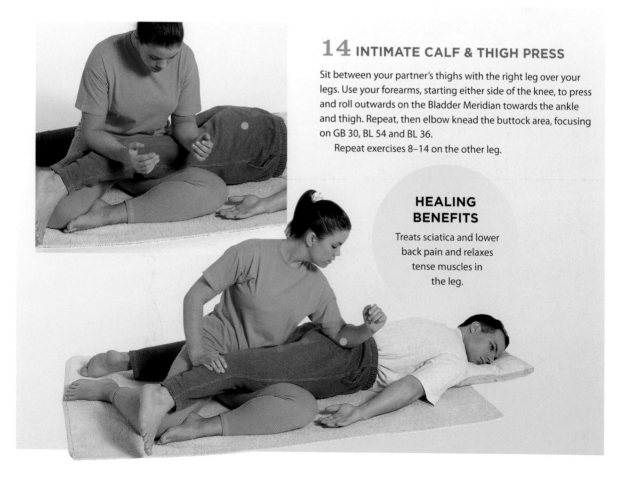

14 INTIMATE CALF & THIGH PRESS

Sit between your partner's thighs with the right leg over your legs. Use your forearms, starting either side of the knee, to press and roll outwards on the Bladder Meridian towards the ankle and thigh. Repeat, then elbow knead the buttock area, focusing on GB 30, BL 54 and BL 36.

Repeat exercises 8–14 on the other leg.

HEALING BENEFITS

Treats sciatica and lower back pain and relaxes tense muscles in the leg.

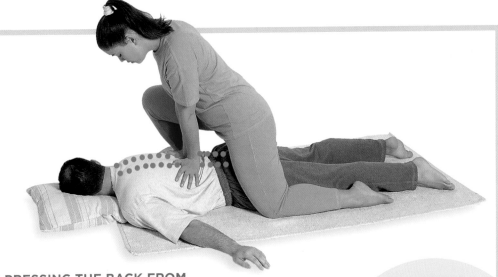

15 PRESSING THE BACK FROM A KNEELING POSITION

Touch method one: palmar pressing (above)

Kneel on one leg astride your partner. With your palm heels on either side of the spine, use both hands to palm deeply and slowly up and down the Sen/Bladder Meridian of the back, between the sacro-lumbar and upper thoracic regions, as shown. Keep your arms straight and use your body weight to generate the required pressure. Finish off by palming the arms.

Touch method two: thumb pressing (above)

Starting with BL 26 bilaterally, thumb press each of the Bladder points located two finger-widths from the midline of the spine on the Sen/Inner Bladder Meridian.

Touch method three: elbow pressing

Repeat the above with elbow pressing on each side.

HEALING BENEFITS

Stimulates energy flow through the back. Releases tense and fibrotic fascia around back muscles and eases lumbago, sciatica and pain due to a slipped disc.

Improves energy flow through the back and all the organs affected by the Bladder Meridian.

Touch method four (below)

This is a variation on touch method one, where you kneel on the back of the thighs just below the buttocks to palmar or thumb press the whole back.

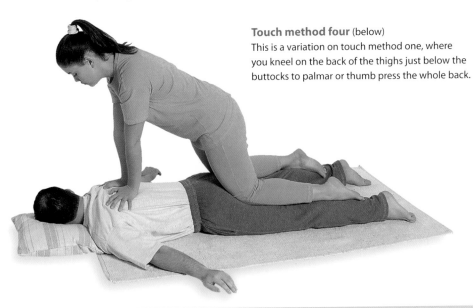

MUSCLES STRETCHED & PRESSED

15 Pressing the back from a kneeling position
Pressed: ERECTOR SPINAE, TRAPEZIUS, RHOMBOIDEUS
MINOR & MAJOR, QUADRATUS LUMBORUM

16 Kneeling cushion cobra
Stretched: PECTORALIS MAJOR, DELTOIDS, RECTUS
ABDOMINIS, PSOAS, ILIACUS, SERRATUS ANTERIOR
Pressed: HAMSTRINGS

CAUTION

Take care when carrying
out the 'cobra' exercises. There should
be no trace of jerkiness in the movements
as these must, at all times, be smoothly
executed for safety reasons.
Many people will experience real discomfort if you
attempt to raise their shoulders more than an inch
or so from the mat. This stretch should only be
performed on those who are fit and fairly flexible.
Don't attempt any of the 'cobra' techniques
on partners heavier than yourself, on the
elderly or those with intervertebral
disc problems.

16 KNEELING CUSHION COBRA

Kneeling on your partner's thighs, grasp the wrists and
ask the receiver to grasp your own wrists. Lean back
and use your weight to lift the upper body into a 'cobra'
position. Hold for at least ten seconds.

Modern living provides few opportunities for
backwards flexion of the spine. To ensure that your
partner's spine remains healthy and pain-free, you must
do both forwards and backwards flexions. (See page 132
for the healing benefits of this exercise.)

17 SITTING STOOL COBRA

Touch method one

Flex your partner's lower legs to 90° so that the soles of the feet are pointing upwards. Sit down carefully on the feet and support your main body weight on your own feet. Palm press the back as described in exercise 15. Lift your partner's arms back and place the wrists across the tops of your thighs. Bend forwards, place your hands under the front of the shoulders and lift them from the mat, using your body weight as you lean backwards. Hold for thirty seconds. Then repeat twice.

HEALING BENEFITS
STEPS 16, 17 & 18

Strong, sustained backwards flexion exercises the articulating joints and associated muscles between the vertebrae, particularly the lumbar ones. Spinal mobility and flexibility are improved, tension and pain in the lower back and between the shoulder blades is eased, and increased shoulder mobility results. Energy flow in the Sen channels of the back increases.

Touch method two

This time your partner interlocks hands behind the head. Repeat the lift, holding the shoulders as in touch method one or under the armpits.

18 STANDING COBRA

Considerable balance is needed to perform this technique correctly. Stand on your partner with one foot placed on each thigh on BL 36 (inset). Your toes should be directed to point outwards, and the arches of your feet should cover the lower margin of the buttocks. Lean forwards, grasp each other's wrists and, with your arms straight, lean backwards so that your weight is pivoted onto your feet. Slowly lift your partner into a 'cobra' position (below). Backwards flexibility of the spine varies greatly, so care must be taken on the first lift to determine how far you can safely go. Each lift should be sustained for up to sixty seconds. Repeat three times.

CAUTION

Many people will experience real discomfort if you try to raise their shoulders more than an inch or so from the mat. This stretch should only be performed on those who are reasonably flexible. Don't attempt any of the 'cobra' techniques on partners heavier than yourself, on the elderly or those with intervertebral disc problems.

MUSCLES STRETCHED & PRESSED
STEPS 17 & 18

Pressed: HAMSTRINGS
Stretched: PECTORALIS MAJOR, DELTOIDS, TERES MAJOR, RECTUS ABDOMINIS, PSOAS MAJOR, ILIACUS, TRAPEZIUS, INFRASPINATUS, SUPRASPINATUS, SERRATUS ANTERIOR

19 WHEELBARROW

Grasp your partner's ankles and lift the legs while, at the same time, positioning one foot over the sacrum and your toes just touching the lower lumbar area. Apply light pressure only. Give the maximum lift that will stretch the front of your partner's thighs effectively without discomfort. Hold this position for about thirty seconds.

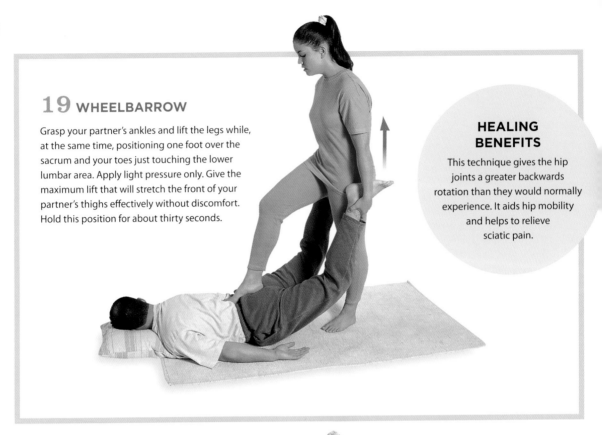

HEALING BENEFITS

This technique gives the hip joints a greater backwards rotation than they would normally experience. It aids hip mobility and helps to relieve sciatic pain.

20 CROSSED AND LATERAL SCISSOR STRETCHES

The methods for these stretches are identical to those used for the lateral and crossed scissor stretches with your partner lying on one side (see page 120), with one exception: the heel of your foot is positioned lightly across the lower spine into BL 25 and BL 26. Repeat on the other side.

CAUTION

This powerful stretch isn't suitable for the elderly or someone with existing back pain.

HEALING BENEFITS

Improves spinal, hip and shoulder flexibility.

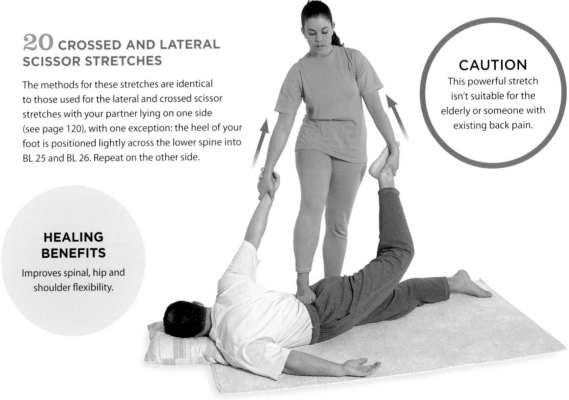

21 KNEE TO CALF PRESS

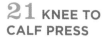

Sit on your partner's sacrum or lumbar region. The exact position is determined by the requirement for your knees to press into the calf muscles. Grasp the front of the ankles and lift them towards you, positioning your knees so that the calf muscles are pulled against them.

HEALING BENEFITS

Relaxes spasming calf muscles and improves energy flow in the lower leg.

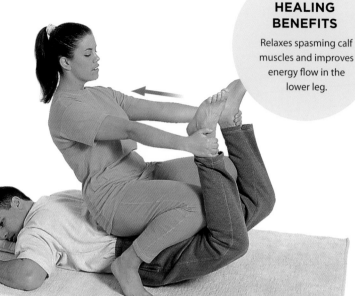

MUSCLES STRETCHED & PRESSED

19 Wheelbarrow
Stretched: PSOAS, ILIACUS, SARTORIUS, RECTUS FEMORIS

20 Crossed & lateral scissor stretches
Stretched: PECTORALIS MAJOR, SARTORIUS, PSOAS MAJOR, ILIACUS
Pressed: ERECTOR SPINAE

21 Knee to calf press
Stretched: QUADRICEPS, PSOAS
Pressed: GASTROCNEMIUS, SOLEUS

22 Intimate cobra
Stretched: PSOAS, ILIACUS, SUPRASPINATUS & INFRASPINATUS, SERRATUS ANTERIOR, PECTORALIS MAJOR, DELTOIDS, RECTUS ABDOMINIS

22 INTIMATE COBRA

Kneel and slide between your partner's thighs, lifting them as you go so that they lie across the front of your hips. Grasp your partner's arms just above the elbow and have your partner grasp your forearms. Lean back with your body weight to lift into the 'cobra' position. Hold for at least ten seconds.

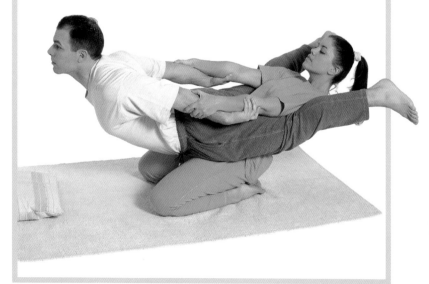

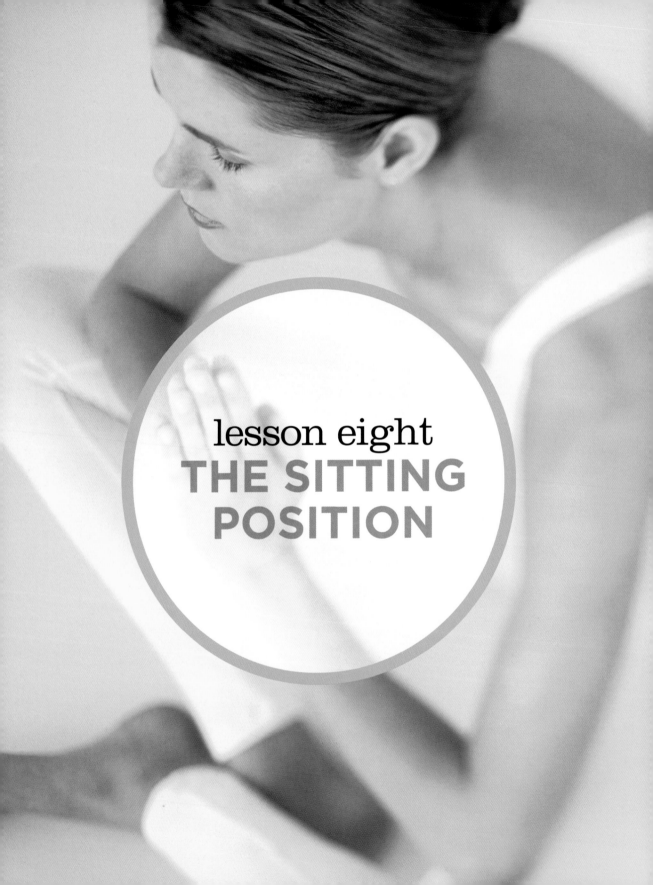

lesson eight
THE SITTING POSITION

Blockages to the flow of energy between the trunk and the head, such as headaches, are released by the techniques used in this part of the bodywork routine. In addition, tense necks and shoulders are relaxed by the pressing and stretching techniques. Some of the exercises are good for treating 'frozen shoulders', and others manipulate the spine. Refer to chapter 2 (see pages 42–51) for the basic pressing and manipulation techniques. The Sen/Meridians shown here represent the upper sections of the Chinese Bladder, Gall Bladder and Small Intestine Meridians. They should be pressed when treating the neck and shoulders in a sitting position.

SEN/MERIDIANS ON THE NECK AND SHOULDERS

Leg Sen 3 Chinese Bladder Meridian Passes just below the base of the skull one finger-width to the side of the midline and passes down either side of the spine between the scapulae.

Leg Sen 2 Chinese Gall Bladder Meridian Passes on either side of the spine in the large depressions immediately below the base of the skull at GB 20 and continues down the top of the shoulders to GB 21.

Hand Sen 3 Chinese Small Intestine Meridian Starts on the outer little finger, passes up the back of the armpit to SI 9, zigzags over the scapula and up the side of the neck.

The Sen/Meridians on the neck and shoulder are:

- **Leg Sen 3 Chinese Bladder Meridian**
- **Leg Sen 2 Chinese Gall Bladder Meridian**
- **Hand Sen 3 Chinese Small Intestine Meridian**

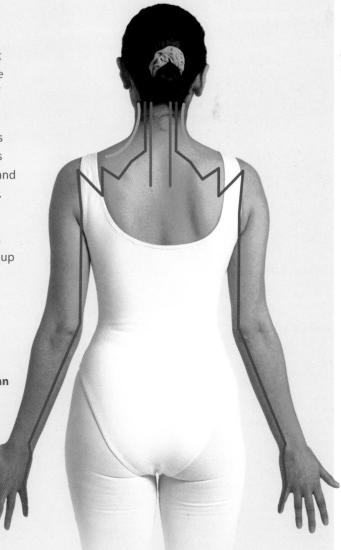

1 PRESSING THE SHOULDERS

Touch method one: palmar pressing

With your palms placed over the top of your partner's shoulders on either side of the neck, press progressively down the shoulders using the heels of your hands. Pressing should be slow and sustained for up to thirty seconds. Gradually increase the pressure by leaning into the presses.

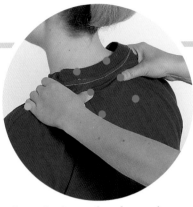

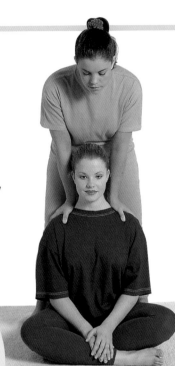

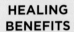

Touch method two: thumb pressing

Thumb press along the tops of your partner's shoulders along the upper scapula and on the soft tissue on either side of the spine on the Bladder Meridian. As you press, feel for any areas of knotted tissue. Strongly knead GB 21 for several minutes.

HEALING BENEFITS

GB 21 relaxes the top of the shoulders and the neck to release daily stress, tension and pain as well as headaches and premenstrual tension.

2 ROLLING THE SHOULDERS WITH THE FOREARMS

Place your forearms on top of your partner's shoulders so that they are positioned directly against the neck and, using your body weight, roll your forearms outwards. Move progressively down to the outer margin of the shoulders. Elbow knead GB 21.

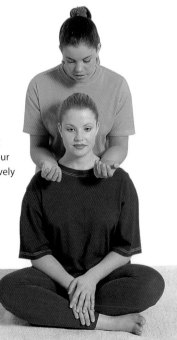

HEALING BENEFITS

This technique reinforces all the benefits of the previous exercise.

MUSCLES STRETCHED & PRESSED

1 **Pressing the shoulders**
   Pressed: TRAPEZIUS, LEVATOR SCAPULAE, ERECTOR SPINAE, RHOMBOIDEUS MAJOR & MINOR

2 **Rolling the shoulders with the forearms**
   Pressed: TRAPEZIUS, LEVATOR SCAPULAE, ERECTOR SPINAE

3 **Thumb pressing the neck**
   Pressed: TRAPEZIUS, SPLENIUS CAPITIS

4 **Interlocked hand/neck press**
   Pressed: ERECTOR SPINAE, LEVATOR SCAPULAE, SPLENIUS CAPITIS

5 **Stretching the neck & shoulders**
   Stretched: STERNOCLEIDOMASTOID

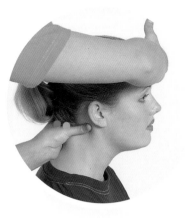

3 THUMB PRESSING THE NECK

Support your partner's forehead lightly with one hand while using the other to thumb and finger press the muscles on either side of the spine. Use a squeezing action. Work from the base of the neck up to the region just below the skull. Knead GB 20 and BL 10. Swap hands to treat the other side. Repeat several times.

HEALING BENEFITS

Releases energy stagnation in the neck. GB 20 relaxes tense neck muscles and relieves headaches and migraines.

4 INTERLOCKED HAND/ NECK PRESS

Tilt your partner's head forwards, interlock the fingers of both hands and thumb press with a pincer-like action up and down the neck on both sides of the spine on the Bladder Meridian. Gradually spread the thumbs to include those muscles that are further away from the midline on the Gall Bladder Meridian.

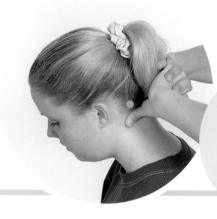

HEALING BENEFITS

Sustained deep pressure relaxes tense muscles, easing pain and stiffness; treats headaches.

5 STRETCHING THE NECK & SHOULDERS

Clasp your hands and place your upper forearm on top of your partner's outer shoulder on GB 21, then carefully position your other forearm against the side of the head just above the ear. Lean your body weight into GB 21 and gently press the head sideways using light pressure on the head. Repeat on the other side.

CAUTION

Take great care not to overstretch the neck. Don't use this technique on the elderly or those with osteoporosis.

HEALING BENEFITS

Stretches the sternocleidomastoid muscles to relieve tension in the sides of the neck.

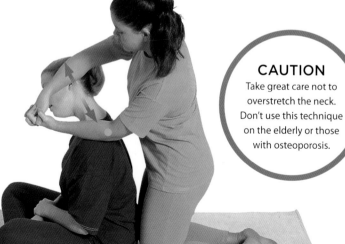

6 BACKWARDS ARM LEVER

Take your partner's left arm, flex it at the
elbow and raise it in a backwards direction,
placing the hand on the left shoulder.
Use your right hand to hold it in position
while your left hand pulls the elbow
backwards. When you feel some resistance
to movement, hold that position for a few
seconds and then release. Repeat on
the other side.

HEALING BENEFITS

Opens the joint
between the scapula
and clavicle. Good for
easing frozen
shoulder.

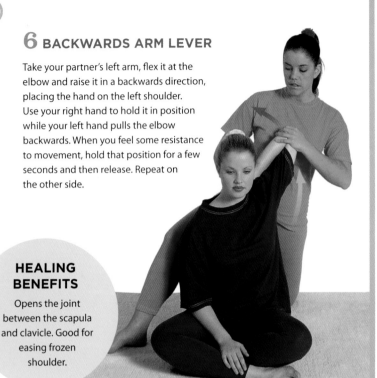

MUSCLES STRETCHED & PRESSED

6 Backwards arm lever
Stretched: PECTORALIS MAJOR, TRICEPS,
LATISSIMUS DORSI, TERES MAJOR &
MINOR, SUBSCAPULARIS

7 Elbow pivot lever
Stretched: PECTORALIS MAJOR,
LATISSIMUS DORSI, SUBSCAPULARIS,
TERES MAJOR & MINOR, DELTOID, TRICEPS,
INFRASPINATUS & SUPRASPINATUS
Pressed: TRAPEZIUS

8 Two-handed hacking on the shoulders
Pressed: TRAPEZIUS

9 Thumbing the shoulders with arm lock
Stretched: PECTORALIS MAJOR
Pressed: INFRASPINATUS &
SUPRASPINATUS

10 Seated lateral arm lever
Stretched: STERNOCLEIDOMASTOID,
TRAPEZIUS, LEVATOR SCAPULAE,
TERES MAJOR & MINOR, ERECTOR
SPINAE, SUBSCAPULARIS, QUADRATUS
LUMBORUM, LATISSIMUS DORSI

7 ELBOW PIVOT LEVER

Raise your partner's left arm and interlock
the fingers with those of your right hand.
Place the back of your elbow very carefully
on the trapezius muscle on top of the
shoulder on GB 21. Lean in with your body
weight. Use this as a pivot as you lift the
elbow backwards with your other hand.
Hold for 30 seconds. Repeat several times
and repeat on the other arm.

HEALING BENEFITS

Aids arm mobility and
eases neck and shoulder
tension and pain.

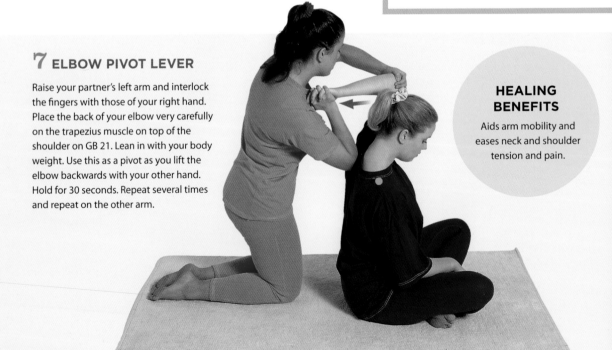

HEALING BENEFITS

Hacking has a soothing effect, leaving the shoulders and upper back feeling very relaxed.

8 TWO-HANDED HACKING ON THE SHOULDERS

Place both your hands lightly together with your fingers spread apart and touching at their tips. Hack across the muscled areas of your partner's shoulders and between the shoulder blades.

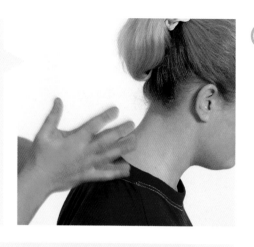

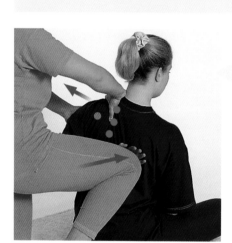

9 THUMBING THE SHOULDERS WITH ARM LOCK

Place your partner's left arm behind the back and hold the hand in position with your right knee. Thumb press up and down the muscled area along the inner border of the shoulder blade on the Bladder Meridian. Knead SI 11. Use your left hand to draw the shoulder back with each thumb press. Repeat on the other arm.

HEALING BENEFITS

Eases neck and shoulder stiffness and pain.

10 SEATED LATERAL ARM LEVER

Kneel with your left knee resting lightly across your partner's thigh. Place the left palm against the side of the head and grasp the elbow. Let the other arm rest across your thigh and grasp the right shoulder so that it's well supported. Now push the left elbow to create strong lateral flexion of the neck and trunk towards the right side. Hold for a few seconds and then repeat this technique on the other side.

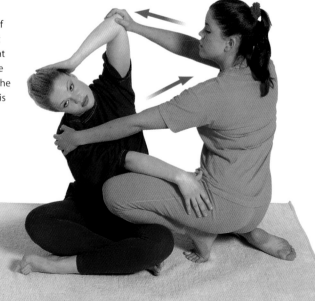

HEALING BENEFITS

Improves lateral flexibility of the spine and eases neck pain and tension. Effectively stretches the muscles down the side of the trunk.

11 SITTING SPINAL TWIST

Using the left arm for support, your partner sits with left leg across the right. Use your left foot to lightly hold the left foot in place. Simultaneously pull your partner's right arm and push the left knee to generate a good spinal twist. Repeat on the other side.

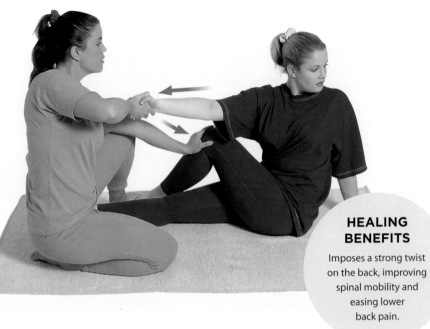

HEALING BENEFITS

Imposes a strong twist on the back, improving spinal mobility and easing lower back pain.

12 PRESSING HEAD TO KNEES

Push your partner's upper body slowly forwards until you feel a point of strong resistance. Flexible subjects will be able to touch their knees with their head. Now palm press and pummel on either side of the spine and the Sen/Bladder Meridian. You can repeat this technique with your partner in the cross-legged position.

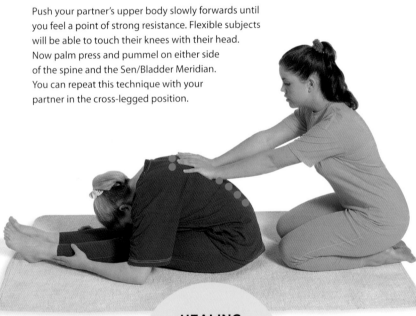

MUSCLES STRETCHED & PRESSED

11 Sitting spinal twist
Stretched: BICEPS, LATISSIMUS DORSI, TRAPEZIUS, RHOMBOIDEUS, PIRIFORMIS, TENSOR FASCIAE LATAE

12 Pressing head to knees
Stretched: ERECTOR SPINAE
Pressed: ERECTOR SPINAE

13 Butterfly shoulder stretch
Stretched: PECTORALIS MAJOR, LATISSIMUS DORSI, TERES MAJOR & MINOR, INFRASPINATUS & SUPRASPINATUS, TRICEPS, DELTOID, SUBSCAPULARIS

14 Butterfly manipulation
Stretched: ERECTOR SPINAE (neck & back), QUADRATUS LUMBORUM

HEALING BENEFITS

Improves forwards flexibility of the spine; invigorates internal organs.

13 BUTTERFLY SHOULDER STRETCH

Ask your partner to clasp the hands behind the neck. Place your forearms against the front of your partner's and then slowly and carefully draw them back to create a strong shoulder stretch. Hold for thirty seconds. Repeat three times.

HEALING BENEFITS

Releases tension in the shoulder muscles and applies a small amount of traction to the upper spine. The joints of the clavicle, sternum and scapula are stretched and shoulder mobility is improved.

14 BUTTERFLY MANIPULATION

Touch method one
With your partner's hands clasped behind the head, tuck your hands under the upper arms and grasp over the clasped hands. Press to guide your partner into a forwards bend in the midline. Hold the position for a few seconds. Repeat several times.

Touch method two
Repeat as above but this time direct your partner's head first towards one knee and then to the other to give a spinal twist.

HEALING BENEFITS

Improves spinal mobility and flexibility, and eases lower back and neck pain and tension.

CAUTION

Don't force your partner beyond the point where resistance is felt. Some people are very stiff when bending in this direction, and only a small degree of flexion is needed.

15 BUTTERFLY SPINAL TWIST MANIPULATION

Retain the same hold on your partner as in the previous technique, but this time place your left knee on the left thigh to hold it in place. Then turn the upper body carefully and slowly to the right to give a powerful spinal twist. Take great care not to overstretch.

HEALING BENEFITS

Gives a twist to the spine and eases lower back pain lateral to the main spinal muscles.

CAUTION

Don't force your partner beyond the point where resistance is felt. Some people are very stiff when twisting sideways, and only a small degree of flexion is needed.

HEALING BENEFITS

Opens the joints between the clavicle and scapula, and also the clavicle and sternum. Energy flow in the channels on either side of the spine is stimulated to ease stiffness and pain in the lower back.

16 FEET TO BACK STRETCH

Sit behind your partner and grasp their wrists. Place your feet on the back on either side of the spine, with your toes level with the lower tips of the shoulder blades. Pull on the arms and press with your feet to create a strong backwards shoulder stretch. You can take tiny alternating steps down the back to the lumbar region.

MUSCLES STRETCHED & PRESSED

15 Butterfly spinal twist manipulation
Stretched: ERECTOR SPINAE (neck & back), QUADRATUS LUMBORUM, LATISSIMUS DORSI, PECTORALIS MAJOR

16 Feet to back stretch
Stretched: PECTORALIS MAJOR, SERRATUS ANTERIOR, RECTUS ABDOMINIS, BICEPS
Pressed: ERECTOR SPINAE

17 Butterfly backwards manipulation
Stretched: ECTORALIS MAJOR, LATISSIMUS DORSI, TERES MAJOR, INFRASPINATUS, RECTUS ABDOMINIS
Pressed: ERECTOR SPINAE

18 Crossed upper arm back manipulation
Stretched: TRICEPS, TRAPEZIUS, RHOMBOIDEUS, SOME ERECTOR SPINAE
Pressed: ERECTOR SPINAE

17 BUTTERFLY BACKWARDS MANIPULATION

Interlock your partner's hands behind their neck, and slide your hands under the armpits, placing your fingers against the forearms. Put your knees against the back just below the shoulder blades and press them into the back against a gentle resistance from your arms. Repeat several times, moving your knees a little further each time.

HEALING BENEFITS

Eases upper back pain, improves flexibility; also relieves tension in the shoulders.

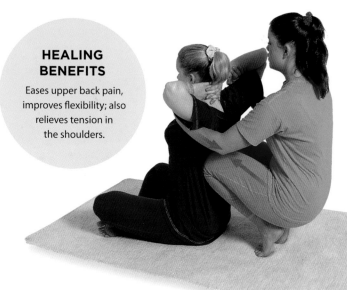

HEALING BENEFITS

Aligns the vertebrae and eases shoulder tension.

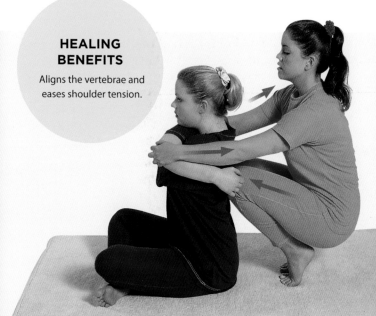

18 CROSSED UPPER ARM BACK MANIPULATION

Cross your partner's arms in front and grasp the right elbow with your left hand and the left elbow with your right hand. Place your knees mid-back on either side of the spine. Pull the elbows until the arms are tight across the chest. Press your knees firmly against your partner. A cracking sound may be heard. Repeat with your knees at different levels.

CAUTION
Don't attempt on the elderly or those with a history of osteoporosis.

TAILOR-MADE TREATMENTS

· · · · · · · · · · · · · · · · · ·

Thai bodywork is used essentially as a form of maintenance to prevent pain, rather than as a means of curing it. Following specific massage routines can, however, soothe some severe areas of discomfort.

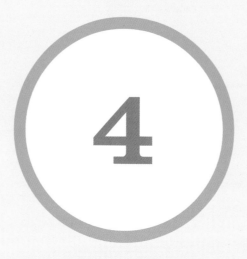

Regular sessions of Thai bodywork can quickly restore good muscle tone and balance between antagonistic groups of muscles. When this has been achieved, the healthy condition is maintained in a way that only the most dedicated yoga practitioner could hope to equal.

The effectiveness of this kind of bodywork is a result of the comprehensive way in which virtually every muscle is treated. None of the muscles – not even the problem ones – can escape attention, provided the full routine for that area is followed.

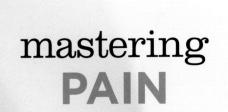

mastering
PAIN

The spine is very much the focal point of Thai massage because a healthy, flexible spine helps to prevent a wide range of chronic pains throughout life. A high proportion of back-pain sufferers have nothing seriously wrong with the structures within their spine. Their problems are due to muscle imbalance around the spine and weak energy flow through them. When tone in the muscles down one side of the backbone is not exactly balanced in the muscles on the other side, postural defects can arise. These soon affect other parts of the body, such as shoulders and hips, and can lead to headaches, sciatica and knee problems.

Expert Thai practitioners are able to treat chronic pain of all kinds; to learn their practices it's advisable to attend a training course. However, for those who learn the art of Thai bodywork through these pages, there are some useful guidelines that can help you handle a partner who suffers from chronic pain such as lower and upper back pain, sciatica, shoulder or neck pain, headaches and hamstring pain. For each of these conditions, a list of the most effective techniques is given. Accompanying diagrams show specific points where extra, sustained pressing is very effective. Treatment focuses strongly on the Bladder Meridian and its points.

MASSAGE ROUTINES TO EASE CHRONIC PAIN

CONDITION	POSITION	THAI MANIPULATIONS
UPPER BACK PAIN This is pain between the shoulder blades. The treatments described here will help to ease this condition.	**1** Prone position	Press the whole back, with emphasis on the area above the waist, for five minutes. Now return to the special points indicated for this region of the back and press deeply for five minutes. • **All the 'cobra' techniques** (pages 131–33, 135)
	2 Supine position	• **Lifting head to straight knees** (page 95)
	3 Side position	• **Rotating the shoulder** (page 114) • **Rotating the shoulder with elbow lever** (page 114) • **Stretching the vertical arm sideways** (page 115) • **Pulling the arm in the side position** (page 116) • **Pulling** and **lifting spinal twists** (page 121) Repeat each of these exercises on the other side of the body.
	4 Seated position	• **Backwards arm lever** (page 140) • **Elbow pivot lever** (page 140) • **Butterfly shoulder stretch** (page 143) • **Feet to back stretch** (page 144) • **Butterfly manipulation** (page 143) • **Crossed upper arm back manipulation** (page 145)
	5 Prone position	Repeat all the presses on the upper back for five minutes.
LOWER BACK PAIN The following routine will help to ease lower back pain.	**1** Prone position	Press the lumbar area either side of the spine for at least five minutes. Pay particular attention to the points marked with a dot.
	2 Supine position	• **Rotating the hips** (page 89) • **Shaking the legs** (page 90) • **Rocking & rolling the back** (page 90) • **The plough** (page 91) • **Rocking the hip** (page 79) • **Shoulder to opposite knee spinal twist** (page 79) • **Stretching the crossed leg horizontally** (page 80) • **Half lotus back rock & roll** (page 82) • **Vertical half lotus thigh press** (page 83) • **Vertical leg stretch** (page 84) • **Bow & arrow spinal twist** (page 89) Repeat each technique on the other leg.
	3 Prone position	Whole back pressing for five minutes. • **Kneeling cushion cobra** (page 131)

CONDITION	POSITION	THAI MANIPULATIONS
LOWER BACK PAIN continued	**3** Prone position (continued)	• **Standing backwards leg lift** (page 126) • **Lateral** and **crossed scissor stretches** (page 120) Repeat pressing of the lower back for five minutes.
	4 Supine position	Repeat the manipulations listed under 2.
SCIATICA These techniques will help with the treatment of sciatica, which results from neuritis of the great sciatic nerve, passing down the back of the thigh.	**1** Prone position	Press the same areas as those indicated for lower back pain (see opposite, below) for five minutes.
	2 Side position	Press the entire outer margin of the flexed leg up to the buttock. Press deeply all around the hip joint, then apply extra pressure to the special points for this area (see below). Press for five to ten minutes, then repeat the pressing on the other leg to balance the back. BOTH SIDES: • **All grape presses** (pages 70–71) • **Shoulder to opposite knee spinal twist** (page 79) • **Knee to knee hip flex** (page 118) • **Stretching the crossed leg horizontally** (page 80) • **Knee pivot hip stretch** (page 119)
	3 Supine position	BOTH LEGS: • **Chest to foot thigh pressing** (page 73) • **Pressing foot to thigh** (page 77) • **Tug of war** (page 78) • **Vertical leg stretch** (page 84) • **Half lotus back rock & roll** (page 82) • **Vertical half lotus thigh press** (page 83) • **Rotating the hips** (page 89) • **The plough** (page 91)

MASSAGE ROUTINES TO EASE CHRONIC PAIN

CONDITION	POSITION	THAI MANIPULATIONS

SHOULDER OR NECK PAIN

Pain in this area of the body is often due to tension. The treatments described here will help.

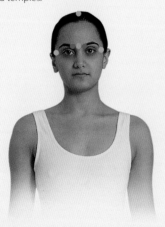

1 Seated position

Press and knead the top of the shoulders. Press the special points deeply for five minutes, gradually increasing the pressure. Press and knead up either side of the neck to just beneath the skull.

- **Backwards arm lever** (page 140)
- **Elbow pivot lever** (page 140)
- **Seated lateral arm lever** (page 141)
- **Feet to back stretch** (page 144)
- **Butterfly shoulder stretch** (page 143)
- **Butterfly manipulation** (page 143)
- **Butterfly backwards manipulation** (page 145)

2 Supine position

- **Pressing the neck** (page 106)
- **Stretching the neck** (page 106)
- **Pulling the turned head** (page 106)
- **Rocking & rolling the back** (page 90)
- **The plough** (page 91)

3 Seated position

Repeat all the neck and shoulder pressing exercises for ten minutes.

HEADACHES

Headaches are caused by energy blockage at the base of the skull and in the forehead and temples.

1 Seated position

Press the neck and shoulders in the same way as for the treatment for neck pain for ten minutes (see above).

2 Supine position

- **Stretching the neck** (page 106)
- **Pulling the turned head** (page 106)
- **Massaging the face and head** (with emphasis on special points) (page 107)

Choose any of the feet techniques from Lesson One (pages 54–63) to bring the energy down.

CONDITION	POSITION	THAI MANIPULATIONS
SORE HAMSTRINGS Sports injury to the hamstrings is common. The following techniques can be used to treat them.	**1** Legs in supine, side and prone positions	• **Palm pressing** (page 46) • **Thumb walking** (page 45)
	2 Supine position	• **Grape presses** (pages 70–71) • **Chest to foot thigh pressing** (page 73) • **Praying mantis** (page 74) • **Pressing foot to thigh** (page 77) • **Tug of war** (page 78) • **Half lotus back rock & roll** (page 82) • **Corkscrew** (page 83) • **Vertical half lotus thigh press** (page 83) • **Raised foot leg stretch** (page 84) • **Vertical leg stretch** (page 84)
	3 Prone position	• **Pressing the thigh & pulling the foot** (page 125) • **Reverse half lotus leg flex** (page 127) • **Intimate calf & thigh press** (page 129) • **Standing cobra** (page 133)
	4 Side position	• **Foot pressing thighs & calves with chair** (page 113)

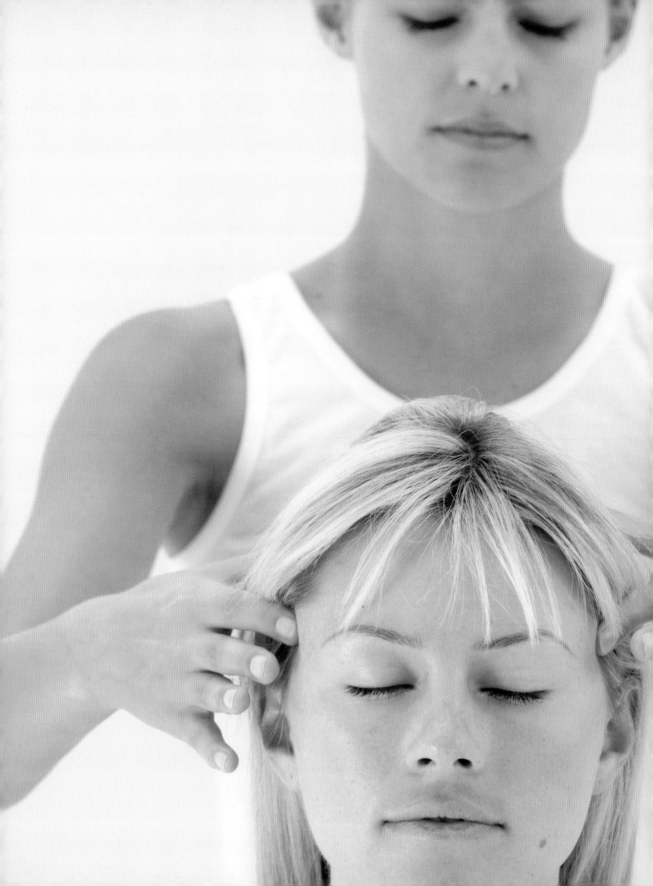

For an absolute beginner, the prospect of having to learn the complete sequence of techniques in this book before carrying out a complete whole-body massage could be daunting. Therefore, we have devised this much-simplified progamme that newcomers should try to master before attempting one that contains all the most advanced techniques.

a programme for
BEGINNERS

RECEIVER LYING ON RIGHT SIDE

PRONE: LEGS & BACK

Repeat steps on the other leg.

SITTING POSITION

INDEX

Page numbers in *italics* refer
to illustrations

RESOURCES

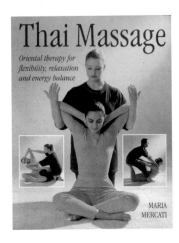

Thai Massage on DVD
by Maria Mercati

This pack of two DVDs is an excellent companion to the *Thai Massage Manual*.

Level 1 – Foundation
Level 2 – Advanced

Training courses

Thai massage, Tui Na Chinese massage and Acupuncture

BODYHARMONICS® CENTRE
54 Flecker's Drive
Hatherley
Cheltenham GL51 5BD
UK
tel: +44 (0)1242 582168

www.bodyharmonics.co.uk
e-mail: maria@bodyharmonics.co.uk

There are very few qualified Thai bodywork therapists in the West. For a register of qualified Thai practitioners in the UK go to: www.acupuncture-acutherapy.co.uk

Further reading

Asokananda (Harald Brust). *The Art of Traditional Thai Massage*, Editions Duang Kamol, 1990

Mercati, Maria. *Step-by-step Tui Na*, Gaia Books, 1997

ACKNOWLEDGEMENTS

I'm indebted to all my teachers in Thailand and in particular to Chaiyuth Priyasith, Songmuang Khanpon, Pramost Wanna, Wandee Boonsai and Praedik to whom I owe a special thank you.

Special thanks go to my husband Trevor for the long hours he devoted to analysing all the main muscles stretched by the Thai techniques, and to my son Graham who studied with me in Thailand. I'm also grateful to him and my daughters Gina and Danella for skilfully demonstrating techniques for the photography, and to my daughter Gisela for promoting Thai massage. Also thanks to my students Alan Orr and Richard Dust, and Shriti Chauhan for additional modelling.

PICTURE CREDITS

Cover India Picture/ShutterStockphoto.Inc

Thinkstock 2 PaaTon; 6 Beboy_ltd; 8 SuratWin; 20 Ryan McVay; 44 Jacek Chabraszewski; 64 George Doyle; 96 George Doyle; 100 Polka Dot Images; 108 George Doyle; 122 George Doyle; 136 Ryan McVay; 148-9 Ryan McVay; 154-5 Stockbyte

ShutterStockphoto.Inc 11 Constantin Stanciu; 54 Piotr Marcinski

iStockphoto 86-7 Nadya Lukic

All other photography by Sue Atkinson

This edition designed and edited by
3REDCARS
www.3redcars.co.uk
for EDDISON BOOKS LIMITED